Map Key

W9-CPZ-127

Other Books of Interest

The Best in Tent Camping: Arizona

The Best in Tent Camping: New Mexico

60 Hikes within 60 Miles: Phoenix

GPS Outdoors: A Practical Guide for Outdoor Enthusiasts

Hikers' and Backpackers' Guide for Treating Medical Emergencies

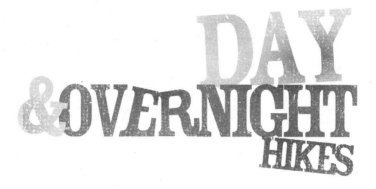

Tonto
National
Forest

TONY PADEGIMAS

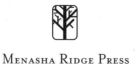

MENASHA RIDGE PRESS

DISCLAIMER

This book is meant only as a guide to select trails in the vicinity of the Tonto National Forest and does not guarantee hiker safety in any way—you hike at your own risk. Neither Menasha Ridge Press nor Tony Padegimas is liable for property loss or damage, personal injury, or death that result in any way from accessing or hiking the trails described in the following pages. Please be aware that hikers have been injured in the Tonto National Forest area. Be especially cautious when walking on or near boulders, steep inclines, and drop-offs, and do not attempt to explore terrain that may be beyond your abilities. To help ensure an uneventful hike, please read carefully the introduction to this book, and perhaps get further safety information and guidance from other sources. Familiarize yourself thoroughly with the areas you intend to visit before venturing out. Ask questions, and prepare for the unforeseen. Familiarize yourself with current weather reports, maps of the area you intend to visit, and any relevant forest service regulations.

Copyright © 2008 by Tony Padegimas
All rights reserved
Published by Menasha Ridge Press
Printed in the United States of America
Distributed by Publishers Group West
First edition, first printing

Text and cover design by Ian Szymkowiak (Palace Press International)
Front cover photograph by Ron Niebrugge/Alamy
Back cover photograph by J. Paul Moore
Author photograph by William M. Kinsey
Cartography and elevation profiles by Scott McGrew and Tony Padegimas
Indexing by Ann Cassar

Library of Congress Cataloging-in-Publication Data

Padegimas, Tony.
    Day & overnight hikes, Tonto National Forest/Tony Padegimas.—1st ed.
      p. cm.
    Includes index.
    ISBN-13: 978-0-89732-639-1
    ISBN-10: 0-89732-639-3
    1. Hiking—Arizona—Tonto National Forest—Guidebooks. 2. Backpacking—Arizona—Tonto National Forest—Guidebooks. 3. Trails—Arizona—Tonto National Forest—Guidebooks. 4. Tonto National Forest (Ariz.)—Guidebooks. I. Title. II. Title: Day and overnight hikes, Tonto National Forest.
    GV199.42.A72T666 2008
    796.5109791—dc22

                            2008030081

Menasha Ridge Press
P.O. Box 43673
Birmingham, Alabama 35243
www.menasharidge.com

Table of Contents

THE HIGH DESERTS

FOUR PEAKS AND MAZATZAL WILDERNESS

THE CENTRAL MOUNTAINS

THE MOGOLLON RIM

About the Author

Tony Padegimas is, among many other things, a freelance writer based alternately in Phoenix, Arizona, or in his hammock strung up in some random spot in the national forest. His wife, two children, and two dogs join him on occasion on the trail but report mixed feelings about whether these endeavors are really worthwhile. The cats have no doubts: they prefer to remain at home in Phoenix.

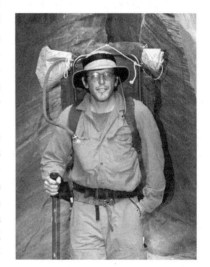

In addition to wanderings in the wilderness, he also chronicles sports, fitness, historical curiosities, technical theatre (which is also his day job), and the inside guts of buildings. His work has appeared in numerous local and regional magazines and a handful of national publications. This is his first book.

Dedication

This book is dedicated to all the hard-working folks, many of them unpaid, who blazed the trails across the rugged wilderness so that we may walk along them simply to amuse ourselves.

Acknowledgments

First and foremost, I must thank all my brave companions who hiked with me, drove to distant trailheads, or waited patiently for me to emerge from the woods. In particular, I would like to thank my wife, my son Ben (who joined more hikes than anyone else), and the rest of my family for juggling things around to make this work possible. I would also like to thank the Rhino Expeditionary Corps, Joe Bartels, and all the fine folks at **HikeAZ.com**—the place to surf when you need advice or companionship for hiking the trails of Arizona.

Preface

This book provides you with an outstanding opportunity to learn from my mistakes. I am not a wilderness expert who happens to be able to write. I am a writer (among many other things) who wanders through the wilderness—just for the fun of it.

I began hiking as a young lad, though my mother, probably more accurately, called it "getting lost in the woods" and secretly hoped I'd take up a more sensible activity. Still, I always wanted to know where the trail actually went, and usually found a way to find out. As I grew older, and kept finding my way back, my mother resigned herself to watching as I walked off on more daring expeditions.

The Tonto National Forest is bigger than you would think. At just under 3 million acres, it is the fifth largest national forest in the United States. Its elevation ranges from 1,300 feet to 7,900 feet, but these numbers only hint at the scale of the place. The mountains aren't particularly big, and the canyons aren't especially deep, but there are a lot of them, and precious little flat land in between.

Much of what is really worth discovering can be reached only by foot. Wilderness boundaries and the sheer ruggedness of the terrain force you to get out of the car and lace up your boots to explore the numerous high peaks, deep gorges, babbling rivers, near-silent deserts, 100-year-old mining camps, or thousand-year-old Native American settlements scattered widely across this multitude of mountains.

Of course, for me, the other part of the challenge is that I get lost—a lot. Some of these trails, some surprisingly easy ones, took two or three attempts because I would get that lost. So when I advise that the narrow trail to the left doesn't go anywhere you want to go, I'm likely speaking from personal experience.

A complete account of the 900 miles of official trails (much less the unofficial trails, trace roads, and bushwhacking routes) would be encyclopedic. This book can only describe a smattering of trails spread out across the Tonto National Forest. I started with a list of 50 hikes that I really wanted to do. That number was whittled down by logistical considerations, fire damage, river levels, and weather to the final 34 described here. Those that made the guide, then, are relatively accessible, though few are easy.

I hiked these trails over eight months with numerous companions, ranging from my 11-year-old son to retired seniors in a local hiking club. My hiking speed, while taking notes, is on the slow end of average—thus the hiking times might be a touch longer than you'll need. A lot of these trails run through canyons where satellite signals are weak to nonexistent. Take all mileages as rough estimates.

There aren't a lot of easy hikes in this forest. All but a handful in this guide are outright adventures. They are all, in my humble opinion, absolutely worth it.

When my mother dropped me off at the Washington Park trailhead (so I could hike the Highline Trail—the last trail I hiked for this guide—back to my car 10 miles to the west), she said that it was still hard for her to watch her little boy (now over 40) walk off by himself into the woods.

She did it anyway. And that, as much as anything else, has made this book possible.

Recommended Hikes

Hikes Good for Dogs

Hikes Good for Swimming

Geology

Hikes Good for Wildflower Viewing

Hikes Good for Seeing Autumn Leaves

Introduction

About this Book

The landscape that is now the Tonto National Forest was born in fire and shaped by water and, to a certain extent, continues to be. The region sits squarely in the Basin and Range geologic province of Arizona—which means there are a lot of mountains separated by a lot of canyons and valleys.

This landscape formed in a slow-motion explosion of magma about 15 million years ago and has been sculpted since by wind and water—mostly water. That water drains into the Salt and Verde watersheds to eventually (if left alone) find the Colorado River.

The Tonto National Forest was specifically created to protect the water that flows into the six large reservoirs formed from dams on the Salt and Verde rivers. There are no natural lakes in the Tonto. Every standing body of water larger than a Jacuzzi has been created by man, from the large reservoirs around Phoenix to the multitude of cattle tanks that dot the remote drainages.

Every year, usually from late May to mid-July, the Forest Service slaps fire restrictions on the entire forest, hoping to prevent, or reduce, the numerous fires that have blackened stretches of landscapes. While fire is somewhat helpful to the lifecycle of a forest, the Sonoran Desert, which stretches into the lower third of the Tonto, does quite well without it. And even in the uplands, uncontrolled fires make life difficult for hikers, among other species.

The hikes in this guide have been organized loosely by climate zone and/or geographic area as follows:

THE LOW DESERTS

Most of these hikes are under 3,500 feet of elevation and are nearest to the Phoenix area. Necessarily short because of the heat and lack of water when crossing the desert, they are among the easiest hikes in the guide.

The Superstition Wilderness

The Superstition Mountain area can be divided into two basic regions: the desert west and the forested east. Much mythology centers on these mountains—long considered home to a vengeful Apache Thunder God and the location of the fabled Lost Dutchman Mine. The range contains a startling variety of rock formations as well as many ruins and relics from Native Americans, cowboys, prospectors, and ranchers.

The High Deserts

Most of these hikes are in the desert at altitudes over 3,500 feet, in a climate zone properly called chaparral. Four of the hikes, including the overnight, are in or near the Cave Creek Trail Complex, north of Carefree, Arizona. The Forest Service supplies an excellent topographical map of this trail system, available at the Cave Creek ranger station.

All of the desert hikes are spectacular in early spring, when the flowers are in bloom. They are difficult, and even dangerous, in the summer, when temperatures can soar above 115°F, even at high altitudes.

Four Peaks and Mazatzal Wilderness

The Four Peaks stand as a sky island in the middle of the desert with the high head of the snake of the Mazatzal Mountains extending northward all the way to the Mogollon Rim. The two hikes on the slopes of Four Peaks are as steep as they are scenic, and worth every calorie burned. The two overnight hikes into nearly opposite corners of the Mazatzal Wilderness are for adventure lovers only.

The Central Mountains

This section includes trails from the Pinal Mountains south of Globe to the foothills of the Mogollon Rim. Mescal Ridge, northeast of Payson, represents the only easy hike in this section. Two hikes loop up and down tall mountains (Pinal and Sierra Ancha), while two plunge down and back up from deep river gorges (Hell's Hole and Hell's Gate).

The Mogollon Rim

This great escarpment defines the northern boundary of the Tonto, as well as the Basin/Range region of the state. Every summer the highway past Payson jams up with desert dwellers rushing to the Rim trying to escape some heat. The 51-mile-long Highline Trail connects numerous side trails, most of which go to or past flowing springs.

How to Use This Guidebook

The Overview Map and Overview-map Key

Use the overview map on the inside front cover to assess the exact locations of each hike's primary trailhead. Each hike's number appears on the overview map, on the map key facing the overview map, and in the table of contents. A hike's full profile is easy to locate as you flip through the book—just look for the hike number at the top of each page.

The book is organized by region, as indicated in the table of contents. The hikes within each region are noted as day hikes or overnight hikes. I have called the out-and-back hikes *trails* and the loop hikes *loops*. For example, "Vineyard Trail" and "Horton Springs Loop."

Trail Maps

Each hike contains a detailed map that shows the trailhead, the route, significant features, facilities, and topographic landmarks such as creeks, overlooks, and peaks. I gathered map data by carrying a GPS (Global Positioning Systems) unit (Garmin Etrex series) while hiking. This data was downloaded into a digital mapping program (Topo USA) and processed by expert cartographers to produce the highly accurate maps found in this book. Each trailhead's GPS coordinates are included with each profile (see below).

Elevation Profiles

Corresponding directly to the trail map, there is a detailed elevation profile with each hike description. The elevation profile provides a quick look at the trail from the side, enabling you to visualize how the trail rises and falls. Key points along the way are labeled. Note the number of feet between each tick mark on the vertical axis (the height scale). To avoid making flat hikes look steep and steep hikes appear flat, height scales are used throughout the book to provide an accurate image of the hike's climbing difficulty.

GPS Trailhead Coordinates

To collect accurate map data, each trail was hiked with a handheld GPS unit (Garmin Etrex series). The data was then downloaded and plotted onto a digital USGS topo map. In addition to rendering a highly specific trail outline, this book also includes the GPS coordinates for each trailhead in two formats: latitude and longitude and Universal Transverse Mercator (UTM). Latitude and longitude coordinates tell you where you are by locating a point west (latitude) of the 0° meridian line that passes through Greenwich, England, and north or south of the 0° (longitude) line that belts the Earth, a.k.a. the equator.

Topographic maps show UTM grid lines in addition to latitude and longitude. Known as UTM coordinates, the numbers index a specific point using a grid method. The survey datum used to arrive at the coordinates in this book is WGS84 (versus NAD27 or WGS83). For readers who own a GPS unit, whether handheld or onboard a vehicle, the latitude and longitude or UTM coordinates provided on the last page of each hike may be entered into the GPS unit. Just make sure your GPS unit is set to navigate using WGS84 datum. Now you can navigate directly to the trailhead.

Most trailheads begin in parking areas, but some hikes require you park then walk a short way to the trailhead. In those cases you'll need a handheld unit if you want to navigate by GPS. That said, readers can easily access all trailheads in this book by using the directions given, the overview map, and the trail map, which shows at least one major road leading into the area. But for those who enjoy using the latest GPS technology to navigate, the necessary data has been provided. A brief explanation of the UTM coordinates for Picketpost Mountain Trail (page 115) follows.

UTM Zone	12S
Easting	483542.25
Northing	3681501.66

The UTM zone number (12) refers to one of the 60 vertical zones of the UTM projection. Each zone is 6 degrees wide. The UTM zone letter (S) refers to one of the 20 horizontal zones that span from 80 degrees south to 84 degrees north. The easting number (483542.25) indicates in meters how far east or west a point is from the central meridian of the zone. Increasing easting coordinates on a topo map or on your GPS screen indicate that you are moving east; decreasing easting coordinates indicate you are moving west. The northing number (3681501.66) references in meters how far you are from the equator. Above and below the equator, increasing northing coordinates indicate you are traveling north; decreasing northing coordinates indicate you are traveling south.

To learn more about how to enhance your outdoor experiences with GPS technology, refer to *GPS Outdoors: A Practical Guide for Outdoor Enthusiasts,* by Russell Helms (Menasha Ridge Press).

THE HIKE PROFILE

In addition to maps, each hike contains a concise but informative narrative of the hike from beginning to end. This descriptive text is enhanced with at-a-glance ratings and information, GPS-based trailhead coordinates, and accurate driving directions that lead you from a major road to the parking area most convenient to the trailhead.

At the top of the section for each hike is a box that allows the hiker quick access to pertinent information: quality of scenery, condition of trail, appropriateness for children, difficulty of hike, quality of solitude expected, hiking distance, approximate hiking time, and outstanding highlights of the trip. The first five categories are rated using a five-star system. Below is an example:

1 Picketpost Mountain

SCENERY: ✦ ✦ ✦ ✦ ✦
TRAIL CONDITION: ✦ ✦
CHILDREN: ✦
DIFFICULTY: ✦ ✦ ✦ ✦
SOLITUDE: ✦ ✦

DISTANCE: *4.45 miles*
HIKING TIME: *4.5 hours*
OUTSTANDING FEATURES: *Big and weird cacti, extraordinary views, cool rock formations, and a little red mailbox full of thoughts.*

The five stars indicate the scenery is very picturesque. The trail condition is fair (one star would mean the trail is likely to be muddy, rocky, overgrown, or otherwise compromised). The one-star rating denotes that only the most gung-ho and physically fit children should go. The four stars for difficulty indicate it is a relatively tough hike (five stars would indicate it's strenuous). You can expect to encounter quite a few people on the trail (with one star you may well be elbowing your way up the trail).

Distances given are absolute, but hiking times are based on an average hiking speed of 2 to 3 miles per hour, with time built in for pauses at overlooks and brief rests. Overnight-hiking times account for the effort of carrying a backpack.

Following each box is a brief description of the hike. A more detailed account follows, in which trail junctions, stream crossings, and trailside features are noted, along with their distance from the trailhead. Flip through the book, read the descriptions, and choose a hike that appeals to you.

Weather

Because of its wide geographic area and great range of altitudes, the Tonto National Forest can see everything from subzero temperatures with snowdrifts to heat of 115°F with single-digit humidity. It is, however, relatively warm and dry throughout most of the national forest most of the time. But this general lack of humidity allows for precipitous drops in temperature once the sun sets.

For weather purposes, the Tonto can be broken up into two basic regions: deserts and highlands.

The Sonoran Desert is infamously hot and dry in the summer but cool and dry in the winter. While daytime highs in the summer can top 115°F, they hover in the 60s and 70s in winter. Overnight lows in summer rarely drop below comfortable room temperature but can plummet below freezing in the winter, especially in the higher deserts.

Parts of the desert get less than eight inches of rain a year, but when it does rain, it comes down hard. Flash flooding can fill a dry wash with a wall of water in minutes.

The central highlands, averaging about 5,500 feet elevation, lack the extremes of the highest and lowest altitudes. With summer highs over 90°F, you will still feel the sun as you climb that hill. And with winter lows in the 20s, you can expect a dusting of snow, and a frozen water bottle, when you wake up in the morning. Year-round, expect a 30°F swing between daytime-high and overnight-low temperatures.

Both regions get their heaviest rainfall in late winter, typically around March, and during the monsoon season, which runs from mid-July through September. During these stretches, storms can appear at any time (especially during monsoon season, when they roll in quite quickly).

If you check the Internet for the weather for Apache Junction or Fountain Hills, you'll get a good idea of prevailing conditions in the desert. Use either Globe or Payson for conditions in the mid-altitude highlands. While there are a number of hikes above 6,000 feet in the Tonto, there are no settlements at that altitude. A good rule is to chop 3°F off the expected temperature per 1,000 feet of elevation gain.

The charts below show the weather for the three distinct elevations of the Tonto National Forest: Low Desert (at around 1,700' elevation), High Desert (at 3,500' elevation), and Highlands (at 5,500' elevation). All temperatures are mean temperatures for that time period in degrees Fahrenheit. All precipitation is shown as mean inches of rain or snow for the given time period. The charts are based on information from the Tonto National Forest Web site.

TEMPERATURE AND PRECIPITATION

Low Desert

	High	Low	Precipitation	Snow
Jan.	65	40	0.6"	0"
Feb.	70	45	0.7"	0"
March	71	45	1.55"	0"
April	80	48	0.2"	0"
May	93	60	0.3"	0"
June	100	70	0.1"	0"
July	105	80	0.2"	0"
Aug.	102	75	1.1"	0"
Sept.	95	72	1.8"	0"
Oct.	88	58	0.4"	0"
Nov.	73	45	1.0"	0"
Dec.	65	40	0.7"	0"

Temperature and Precipitation

High Desert

	High	Low	Precipitation	Snow
Jan.	59	30	1.45"	1.2"
Feb.	62	35	1.0"	0.5"
March	65	38	1.5"	0.6"
April	77	44	0.5"	0"
May	85	50	0.3"	0"
June	95	58	0.3"	0"
July	97	68	2.3"	0"
Aug.	95	65	2.8"	0"
Sept.	91	59	1.5"	0"
Oct.	82	47	1.3"	0"
Nov.	68	38	0.8"	0.2"
Dec.	59	32	1.7"	0.4"

Temperature and Precipitation

Highlands

	High	Low	Precipitation	Snow
Jan.	50	22	2.5"	9.5"
Feb.	53	23	2.3"	10"
March	58	25	2.4"	12.5"
April	63	29	1.0"	2.9"
May	73	35	0.3"	0.1"
June	84	42	0.4"	0"
July	87	52	3.8"	0"
Aug.	84	52	4.2"	0"
Sept.	78	45	2.05"	0"
Oct.	71	36	2.1"	0.3"
Nov.	59	28	2.1"	4.6"
Dec.	55	24	3.1"	12.5"

Lightning

The Mogollon Rim claims the most lightning strikes of any spot in federal lands. During the monsoon season (July through September), try to reach high-altitude summits by 1 p.m. and retreat if the weather turns bad. If you are caught in a lightning storm, stay off ridgetops, spread out (if you are in a group), and squat or sit on a foam pad with your feet together. Keep away from rock outcroppings and isolated trees. If someone has been struck, be prepared to use CPR to help restore their breathing and heartbeat.

Hyperthermia

Hyperthermia occurs when your core body temperature becomes dangerously high. This can happen with alarming speed when the sun is hot and shade and water are in short supply. It is a particular hazard when climbing uphill. Hyperthermia manifests in two particular conditions: heat exhaustion and heatstroke. Heat exhaustion is typically triggered by dehydration. Symptoms include heavy sweating, paleness, dizziness, headache, muscle cramps, and a high temperature. The remedy is to cool off: get in the shade, drink plenty of cool fluids, and remove as many layers of clothing as practical. Stay in the shade until the symptoms are gone.

Trying to power through heat exhaustion can lead to heatstroke—which not only ends your hike but has a fair chance of ending your life if not treated. The chief warning sign of heatstroke (besides the symptoms of heat exhaustion) is that you stop sweating. If you're hot and you are not sweating, that's big trouble, and you need to fix it right now. Heatstroke is a life-threatening condition that causes seizures, convulsions, and eventually death. Do whatever can be done to cool the victim down, and seek medical attention as soon as possible.

Hypothermia

Hypothermia occurs when your core body temperature is dangerously low. You can suffer this at any time of the year, and cold temperatures, wind, rain, and snow set the stage for complications. Look for signs of shivering, loss of coordination, and impaired judgment. Prevention in the form of preparation is your best defense against getting cold to the core. Remember the mantra "wet is not warm" to prevent hypothermia. Keep your inside layer as dry as possible.

Water

How much is enough? One simple physiological fact should convince you to err on the side of excess when deciding how much water to pack: A hiker working hard in 90° heat needs approximately ten quarts of fluid per day. That's 2.5 gallons—12 large water bottles or 16 small ones. Pack along one or two bottles even for short hikes.

For most people, the pleasures of hiking make carrying water a relatively minor price to pay to remain healthy. A good reason to carry all your water is that springs and streams are notoriously unreliable throughout the Tonto, particularly in the deserts, where depending upon a spring could prove to be a fatal gamble.

Probably the most common waterborne "bug" that hikers face is giardia, which may not hit until one to four weeks after ingestion. It will have you living in the bathroom, passing noxious rotten-egg gas, vomiting, and shivering with chills. Other parasites to worry about include E. coli and cryptosporidium, both of which are harder to kill than giardia.

Some hikers and backpackers hit the trail prepared to purify water found along the route. This method, while less dangerous than drinking it untreated, comes with risks. Purifiers with ceramic filters are the safest. Many hikers pack the slightly distasteful tetraglycine-hydroperiodide tablets to debug water (sold under the names Potable Aqua, Coughlan's, and others). These can make pure spring water taste like city tap—but they are effective at killing the nasties. Or if you have the means and the time, bringing found water to a rolling boil for at least two minutes kills everything.

If you're tempted to drink found water, do so only if you understand the risks. Better yet, hydrate before your hike, carry (and drink) six ounces of water for every mile you plan to hike, and hydrate after the hike.

The Ten Essentials

One of the first rules of hiking is to be prepared for anything. The simplest way to be prepared is to carry the "Ten Essentials." In addition to carrying the items listed below, you need to know how to use them, especially navigation items. Always consider worst-case scenarios such as getting lost, hiking back in the dark, having gear break (for example, breaking a hip strap on your pack or having a water filter get plugged up), twisting an ankle, or encountering a brutal thunderstorm. The items listed below don't cost a lot of money, take up much room in a pack, or weigh much, but they might just save your life.

WATER: durable bottles and water treatment such as iodine
   or a filter

MAP: preferably a topo map and a trail map with a route description

COMPASS: a high-quality compass

FIRST-AID KIT: a good-quality kit with first-aid instructions

KNIFE: a multitool device with pliers is best

LIGHT: flashlight or headlamp with extra bulbs and batteries

FIRE: windproof matches or lighter and fire starter

EXTRA FOOD: you should always have food in your pack when you've
   finished hiking

EXTRA CLOTHES: rain protection, warm layers, gloves, warm hat

SUN PROTECTION: sunglasses, lip balm, sunblock, sun hat

First-aid Kit

A typical first-aid kit may contain more items than you might think necessary. The ones in the list that follows are just the basics. Prepackaged kits in waterproof bags (Atwater Carey and Adventure Medical make a variety of kits) are available. Even though quite a few items are listed below, they pack down into a small space:

Ace® bandages or Spenco® joint wraps

Antibiotic ointment (Neosporin® or the generic equivalent)

Athletic tape

Band-Aids®

Benadryl® or the generic equivalent diphenhydramine (in case of allergic reactions)

Butterfly-closure bandages

Electrical tape (holds bandages in place rain or shine)

Epinephrine in a prefilled syringe (for people known to have severe allergic reactions to such things as bee stings; usually by prescription only)

Gauze (one roll)

Gauze compress pads (a half dozen 4 x 4–inch pads)

Hydrogen peroxide or iodine

Ibuprofen or acetaminophen

Insect repellent

Moleskin/Spenco 2nd Skin®

Sunscreen

Superglue (bonds skin instantly, if all else fails)

Tweezers

The following items are optional but worth their weight:

Aluminum foil

Bandana

Carabiners

Cellular phone (emergencies only)

Dark chocolate (at least 60% cocoa)

Digital camera

Disinfectant wipes

Extra batteries

Foam pad (for lightning strikes)

Garbage bag

Gloves (for warmth)

GPS receiver

Lip balm

Matches or pocket lighter

Plastic bags with zip closure

Raincoat and rain pants

Toilet paper

Watch

Whistle (more effective in signaling rescuers than your voice)

General Safety

· DO NOT EVER RELY ON CELL PHONES IN THE TONTO NATIONAL FOREST. Signals and access are very inconsistent. Check with your cellular service provider before leaving home. Many outdoor enthusiasts rely on GPS and other forms of communication in the backcountry. Even this can be inconsistent in the deeper canyons.

· ALWAYS CARRY FOOD AND WATER, whether you are planning to go overnight or not. Food will give you energy, help keep you warm, and sustain you in an emergency situation until help arrives. You never know if you will have a stream nearby when you become thirsty. In the desert, water sources can be unreliable or completely nonexistent. Bring potable water or boil or filter all found water before drinking it.

· STAY ON DESIGNATED TRAILS. Most hikers get lost when they leave the path. Even on the most clearly marked trails, there is usually a point where you have to stop and consider which direction to head. If you become disoriented, don't panic. As soon as you think you may be off track, stop, assess your current direction, and then retrace your steps to the point where you went astray. Using a map, compass, and this book, keep in mind what you have passed to that point, reorient yourself, and trust your judgment on which way to continue. If you become absolutely unsure of how to continue, return to your vehicle the way you came in. Should you become completely lost and have no idea how to return to the trailhead, remaining in place along the trail and waiting for help is most often the best option for adults and always the best option for children.

- BE ESPECIALLY CAREFUL WHEN CROSSING STREAMS. Whether you are fording the stream or crossing on a log, make every step count. If you have any doubt about maintaining your balance on a log, ford the stream instead. When fording a stream, use a trekking pole or stout stick for balance and face upstream as you cross. If a stream seems too deep to ford, turn back. Whatever is on the other side is not worth risking your life.

- BE CAREFUL CLIMBING UP AND DOWN. Be prepared to use the sides of your boots, or even your butt, if necessary, to control your descent down steep grades. In many places, once you start tumbling down, you won't stop for a long time. When climbing a steep incline, know your limits. Remember, you may have to get down this way, too. Don't blindly assume the decomposing granite or basalt outcropping will hold your weight. When climbing with a group, be aware that the chunk of basalt that crumbled beneath your feet is going to keep falling. Leave each other some distance.

- LOOK UP, when choosing a spot to rest or a backcountry campsite. Standing dead trees (common in fire zones) and storm-damaged living trees may have loose or broken limbs that could fall at any time.

- TAKE ALONG YOUR BRAIN. A cool, calculating mind is the single most important piece of equipment you'll ever need on the trail. Think before you act. Watch your step. Plan ahead. Avoiding accidents before they happen is the best strategy for a rewarding and relaxing hike.

- ASK QUESTIONS. Tonto Forest rangers are there to help. It's a lot easier to get advice beforehand and avoid a mishap than to amend an error after you're away from civilization and it's too late. Use your head out there and take care of the place as if it were your own backyard.

Mineshafts

Many areas in the Tonto have been extensively mined, often by tunneling. These tunnels are holes in the ground where holes should not be, and climbing into them places more faith in the engineering acumen of whatever prospector dug this 100 years ago than is perhaps wise. Also, they are excellent breeding grounds for all manner of vermin. Moreover, the Sierra Ancha area was extensively mined for uranium before it was designated a wilderness area, so those holes are potentially radioactive as well. Stay out of them.

Animal and Plant Hazards

The Tonto National Forest has all sorts of wildlife: mule deer, bighorn sheep, coyote, elk, javelina, ring-tailed cats, and more. Here's a quick primer on how best to enjoy watching wildlife:

- Never, ever feed wildlife.

- Watch from a distance.

- Obey all closure signs.

- Drive cautiously and do not block traffic to look at wildlife.

BLACK BEARS

While rare, black bears are known to wander the more remote portions of the Tonto. There are no definite rules about what to do if you meet a bear. In most cases the bear will detect you first and leave. If you do encounter a bear, here are some suggestions from the National Park Service:

- Stay calm.

- Move away, talking loudly to let the bear discover your presence.

- Back away while facing the bear.

- Avoid eye contact.

- Give the bear plenty of room to escape; bears will rarely attack unless they are threatened or provoked.

- Don't run or make sudden movements; running will provoke the bear, and you cannot outrun it.

- Do not attempt to climb trees to escape bears, especially black bears. The animal will pull you down by the foot.

- Fight back if attacked. Black bears have been driven away when people have fought back with rocks, sticks, binoculars, and even their bare hands.

Mountain Lions

Lion attacks on people are rare, with fewer than 12 fatalities in 100 years. Based on observations by people who have come in contact with mountain lions, some patterns are beginning to emerge. Here are more suggestions from the National Park Service:

- Stay calm.

- Talk firmly to the lion.

- Move slowly.

- Back up or stop; never run—lions will chase and attack.

- Raise your arms. If you are wearing a sweater or coat, open it and hold it wide.

- Pick up children to make them appear larger.

- If the lion becomes aggressive, throw rocks and large objects at it. This is the time to convince the lion that you are not prey and that you are a danger to them.

- Never crouch or turn your back to retrieve items.

- Fight back and try to remain standing if you are attacked.

Ticks

Ticks like to hang out in the brush that grows along trails. Their numbers seem to explode in the hot summer months, but you should be tick-aware year-round. Ticks, which are arthropods and not insects, need to feast on a host in order to reproduce. The ticks that light onto you while you hike will be very small, sometimes so tiny that you won't be able to spot them. Primarily of two varieties, deer ticks and dog ticks, ticks need a few hours of attachment before they can transmit any disease they may harbor. Ticks may first settle in shoes, socks, or hats, and may take several hours to latch on to your person. The best strategy is to visually check every half hour or so while hiking, do a thorough check before you get in the car, and then, when you take a post-hike shower, do an even more thorough check of your entire body. Ticks that haven't attached are easily removed but not easily killed. If you pick off a tick in the woods, just toss it aside. If you find one on your body at home, dispatch it and then send it down the toilet. For ticks that have embedded, removing them with tweezers is best.

SNAKES AND GILA MONSTERS

Rattlesnakes are common in the Tonto, whereas Gila monsters are still somewhat rare. Nevertheless, I encountered both while preparing the guide. These reptiles have the right-of-way. The best advice is to give them a wide berth and let them move away from you (which can be time-consuming with Gila monsters). In the event that you are bitten by a rattlesnake, stay calm and get help immediately.

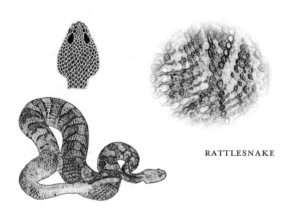

RATTLESNAKE

There's not much you can do in the field that's not going to make it worse. Get out and get help.

Although rattlesnakes can be found throughout the Tonto, the Gila monster is found only in the desert areas. Their bite is not nearly as venomous, but they like to clamp down and hold on, which will hurt—a lot. And you will need medical attention. Gila monsters are heavily protected by state law. Don't shoot them.

Cacti

Numerous species of these spiny succulents are found all over the Tonto, right up to the 6,000-foot line. While all of them are capable of jabbing you on contact, the various species of cholla or jumping cacti are by far the biggest threat. You need only brush it slightly for the numerous, sharp spines to go into your skin, and then curl up inside, making their removal difficult and painful.

Wear good boots and watch where you put your hands. If you do get nailed, you need to pull the spines out. A fine-toothed comb can sometimes be used to remove the smaller spines, but for bigger ones you'll need a good set of tweezers. Keep one in your first-aid kit. Take care that the remaining puncture wounds do not become infected.

A related menace, especially at middle altitudes, is the acacia catclaw, a nasty little shrub with razor-sharp thorns that greedily shred any flesh or gear passing through them. In catclaw country, keep spare clothing and inflatables inside your pack. Some hikers wear thick gaiters or even soccer guards when hiking through the transition scrub where this species can be dominant.

Poison Ivy

Recognizing poison ivy and avoiding contact with it is the most effective way to prevent the painful, itchy rashes associated with this plant. Urushiol, the oil in the sap of poison ivy, is responsible for the rash. Usually within 12 to 14 hours of exposure (but sometimes much later), raised lines and/or blisters will appear, accompanied by

INTRODUCTION

COMMON POISONOUS PLANTS

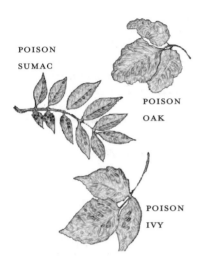

POISON SUMAC

POISON OAK

POISON IVY

a terrible itch. Refrain from scratching because bacteria under fingernails can cause infection and you will spread the rash to other parts of your body. Wash and dry the rash thoroughly, applying calamine lotion or another product to help dry the rash. If itching or blistering is severe, seek medical attention. Remember that oil-contaminated clothes, pets, or hiking gear can also cause the rash, so wash not only any exposed parts of your body but also clothes, gear, and pets.

Mosquitoes

Although it's not common, individuals can become infected with the West Nile virus by being bitten by an infected mosquito. Culex mosquitoes, the primary variety that transmits West Nile virus to humans, thrive in urban rather than natural areas. They lay their eggs in stagnant water and can breed in any standing water that remains for more than five days. Most people infected with West Nile virus have no symptoms of illness, but some may become sick, usually 3 to 15 days after being bitten.

Anytime you expect mosquitoes to be buzzing around, you may want to wear protective clothing, such as long sleeves, long pants, and socks. Loose-fitting, light-colored clothing is best. Spray clothing with insect repellent. Remember to follow the instructions on the repellent and to take extra care with children.

Tips for Enjoying Tonto National Forest

- Visit the Tonto National Forest Web site: **http://www.fs.fed.us/r3/tonto/ home.shtml** for information about facilities, access, and any fire and flood closures. Click on Recreational Activities and then Hiking and Trailriding to find information (which ranges from a vague paragraph to a complete pamphlet, depending on the hike) on the various trails and trailheads.

- You need a Tonto Pass to use many of the recreation sites nearest to the Phoenix area, particularly around the lakes. A one-day pass costs $6 per vehicle and $4 per watercraft and is available at any ranger station and at a multitude of merchants near the respective recreation areas. Multiday passes are also available. You can also buy a pass online at the Tonto National Forest site listed above. The annual pass has been quietly discontinued, and areas accepting one are dwindling, though it will still be valid at the most common sites.

- Most of the fee areas on or near the Mogollon Rim, particularly the campgrounds, are run by private concessionaires and do not accept Tonto passes. Some take checks; all take cash.

- Of the trailheads listed in this book, only two, Butcher Jones and Rattlesnake Cove (the Palo Verde Trail), require a Tonto pass. All of the other trailheads listed can be used free of charge.

- Forest Roads are maintained on a need-to-use basis, which means some are not maintained at all. Inquire about road conditions before setting out, particularly if it has been raining. There are several trailheads listed in this guide that cannot be reached by wheeled conveyance after heavy rains.

- Many hikes are in wilderness areas that have their own set of rules, the primary one being no wheels. This includes mountain bikes. You are also limited to 15 people in a group and/or 15 head of livestock, if that somehow concerns you.

- Dogs are required to be kept on a leash throughout the national forest.

- The Tonto National Forest reliably applies fire restrictions starting sometime around Memorial Day and extending into July. This means no campfires anywhere and no smoking. Any stove must be able to be instantly extinguished, which leaves, for practical purposes, only liquid fuel stoves.

Tips for a Happy Camping Trip

There is nothing worse than a bad camping trip, especially because it is so easy to have a great time. To assist with making your outing a happy one, here are some pointers:

- ALWAYS STRIVE TO PRACTICE LOW-IMPACT CAMPING. Adhere to the adages "Pack it in, pack it out," and "Take only pictures, leave only footprints." Practice "Leave no trace" camping ethics while in the backcountry.

- PICK YOUR CAMPING BUDDIES WISELY. A family trip is pretty straightforward, but you may want to consider excluding grumpy Uncle Fred, who does not like bugs, sunshine, or marshmallows. After you know who is going, make sure that everyone is on the same page regarding expectations of difficulty, sleeping arrangements, and food requirements. This is doubly important on backpacking expeditions since you can't just pile back into the car if things go sour.

- DON'T DUPLICATE EQUIPMENT such as cooking pots and lanterns among campers in your party. Carry what you need to have a good time, but don't turn the trip into a major moving experience.

- DRESS APPROPRIATELY FOR THE SEASON. Educate yourself on the highs and lows of the specific area you plan to visit. It may be warm at night in the summer in your backyard, but up in the mountains it will be chilly.

- PITCH YOUR TENT ON A LEVEL SURFACE, preferably one that is covered with leaves, pine straw, or grass. Pitch your tent on a tarp or specially designed footprint to thwart ground moisture and to protect the tent floor. Do a little site maintenance, such as picking up small rocks and sticks that can damage your tent floor and make sleep uncomfortable. If you have a separate tent rainfly but don't need it, keep it rolled up at the base of the tent in case it starts raining at midnight.

- TAKE A SLEEPING PAD WITH YOU. Use one that is full-length and thicker than you think you might need. This will not only keep your hips from aching on hard ground but will also help keep you warm.

- IF YOU ARE NOT HIKING INTO A PRIMITIVE CAMPSITE, there is no real need to skimp on food due to weight. Plan tasty meals and bring everything you will need to prepare, cook, eat, and clean up the mess.

Trail and Camping Etiquette

Always remember that great care and resources (from both nature and your tax dollars) have gone into creating these trails. Treat the trail, wildlife, and fellow hikers with respect.

- HIKE ON OPEN TRAILS ONLY.

- LEAVE ONLY FOOTPRINTS. Be sensitive to the ground beneath you. This also means staying on the existing trail and not blazing any new trails. Be sure to pack out what you pack in. No one likes to see the trash someone else has left behind, so be part of the solution and pick that up as well whenever practical.

- NEVER SPOOK ANIMALS. An unannounced approach, a sudden movement, or a loud noise startles most animals. A surprised elk can be dangerous to you, to others, and to itself. Give animals extra room and time to adjust to your presence.

- PLAN AHEAD. Know your equipment, your ability, and the area where you are hiking—and prepare accordingly. Be self-sufficient at all times. Carry necessary supplies for changes in weather or other conditions. A well-executed trip is a satisfaction to you and to others.

- BE COURTEOUS to other hikers or equestrians you meet on the trails.

- OBTAIN ALL PERMITS AND AUTHORIZATIONS AS REQUIRED. Make sure you check in, pay your fee, and mark your site as directed. Don't make the mistake of grabbing a seemingly empty site that looks more appealing than your site. It could be reserved.

- STRICTLY FOLLOW THE RULES REGARDING THE BUILDING OF FIRES. While the Tonto is fairly liberal about campfires through the winter, nothing brings out angry rangers faster than a pillar of smoke during a fire restriction. And you can hardly avoid ample evidence of what can happen if the fire gets out of its circle.

The Low Deserts

1

Explore
numerous
high peaks
deep gorges
babbling
river
beds
near-silent
deserts,
hundred-
year-old
mining
camps,
or thousand-
year-old
Native
American
settlements

SCENERY: ♟ ♟	DISTANCE: *5.25 miles*
TRAIL CONDITION: ♟ ♟ ♟ ♟	HIKING TIME: *2 hours*
CHILDREN: ♟ ♟ ♟ ♟	OUTSTANDING FEATURES: *Views of lake and*
DIFFICULTY: ♟	*surrounding basin, cacti, fishing access*
SOLITUDE: ♟	

This easy hike starts at the Saguaro nature trail and then follows the shore of Saguaro Reservoir around Peregrine Point to Camper's Cove. From there it cuts across a peninsula through some pristine desert to terminate at Burro Cove. A great hike for dogs and kids and other limited hikers. Also provides shoreline access for fishing, or just skipping rocks.

🥾🥾 This hike begins as the Saguaro Lake Nature Trail, with a trailhead from the Butcher Jones Recreation Area parking lot, near the beach. The nature trail portion is wheelchair accessible—except for the very first part, which is a dirt gulley. You could probably get a wheelchair across it, but you'd have to really, really want to. Once past this gulley, though, the trail comes complete with asphalt, railings, and interpretive signs.

One sign points out the various trees found in Arizona riparian areas—but this reservoir, mostly lined with mesquite trees, isn't one of them.

Another sign lists animals you might see: bald eagles, great blue herons, coyotes, ring-tailed cats, and bats. They left out ducks and skunks—which are actually quite common.

The nature trail goes roughly southeast, following the shoreline through the high desert ecology that surrounds the reservoir. So to your left you'll see saguaros, palo verde trees, and buckhorn cholla, but on your right a sea of reeds as tall as you are separates the trail

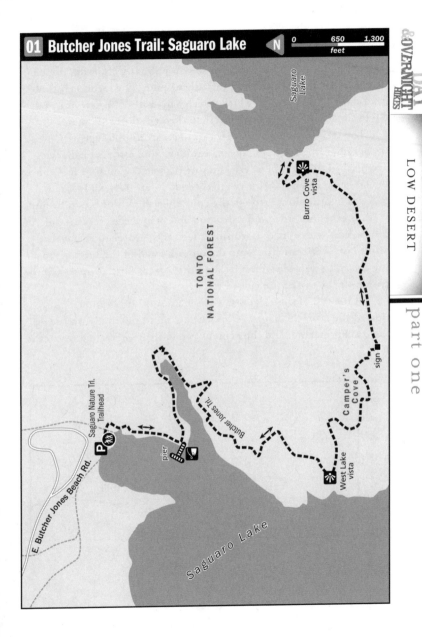

01 Butcher Jones Trail: Saguaro Lake

N

0   650   1,300
feet

DAY & OVERNIGHT HIKES

LOW DESERT

part one

Saguaro Lake

TONTO NATIONAL FOREST

Burro Cove vista

Camper's Cove

sign

West Lake vista

Butcher Jones Trl.

E. Butcher Jones Beach Rd.

Saguaro Nature Trl. Trailhead

P

pier

Saguaro Lake

from the lake. Across the little bay you can see the orange cliffs covered with bright-yellow lichen.

The nature trail portion goes for only about 0.25 miles, terminating in the turnoff to a floating fishing pier. The secondary trailhead starts here, through which wheelchairs will definitely not pass. Go to the left of the railing, and then through the cattle maze.

The trail soon turns sharply east to go around Peregrine Cove, a sizable inlet lined with mesquite, boulders, and assorted fishermen. The packed dirt and powdered granite path stays about 50 feet above the lake. At the end of this relatively deep inlet, the trail U-turns, practically tunneling through the combined thicket of mesquite and reeds on the lake side, and ironwood and palo verde trees on the other. You've dropped to within 12 feet of the water line, but that won't last. The trail climbs up the opposite wall of the inlet, winding around a sizeable side inlet, and then heads farther up to exit the cove near the top of the ridge line.

At the top of the ridge you can see most of the southern portion of the lake, the happy yellow cliffs around Butcher Jones cove, the distant marina, and the grim brown cliffs immediately across the

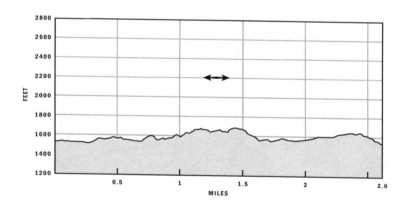

water. From here you can see clearly what a marvelous canyon this must have been before it was flooded. Here you stand at 1,700 feet—the highest point of the hike.

The route goes south from here toward Camper's Cove, with a good hundred feet of steep, cactus-covered slope separating the trail from the water. Even as the trail winds over ridges and around ravines, it still goes easy, and it still goes south.

After the 1.3-mile mark, the trail will begin to go down more often than up as you wander down into Camper's Cove. Barrel and teddy bear cholla cacti become more common with buckhorn cholla appearing less often.

At 1.6 miles, a sign announces Camper's Cove, which is a desert-covered hill that slopes down to a gravelly beach. A short distance past this, another wooden sign will reassert that you are still on Butcher Jones Trail 463, and indicates 0.5 miles to shore access or 0.75 miles to Burro Cove. Go straight, in and out of the steep ravine, toward Burro Cove. (The sign actually uses fractions, none of which are accurate.)

The route now cuts inland, heading east across the peninsula that separates Camper's Cove from Burro Cove, and forms one of the two great turns in the S shape of the reservoir. This portion feels more like real desert. Erosion and gravity have carved some cool rock formations out of the hill that crowns the peninsula. Cholla, acacia, ocotillo, and palo verde trees all crowd the trail through here as if they are pressing in to shake your hand. This is particularly true of the teddy bear cholla, which is infamous for shaking hands whether invited or not.

A second directional sign indicates that you are almost across this micro-desert passage, and soon thereafter you will see the lake in the distance once more.

At 2.5 miles in, you stand at the top of the peninsular ridge, looking over the other half of the S of accumulated water that forms

DAY & OVERNIGHT HIKES

LOW DESERT

part one

Saguaro Reservoir. On a clear day, Four Peaks will be visible across the waters.

Past here the trail turns north and steeply down hill. The path degrades the farther you go. The problem is not so much the surface, which is rocky but passable, but the low mesquite and palo verde branches, which force any creature taller than, well, a burro, to repeatedly duck or bushwhack.

The trail doesn't actually descend to the waterline, but you can get there after another 50 to 100 feet of bushwhacking. The zones radiating out from the water are fairly constant: gravel, reeds, garbage, mesquite, and desert.

When you are finished skipping stones across the water, return the way you came.

DIRECTIONS: From Mesa, take AZ 87 north 27 miles to Bush Highway and turn right. Follow Bush Highway to Forest Road 166. A sign will lead you to the Butcher Jones Recreation Area, 2 miles down FR 166. This site has paved parking, beach access, vault toilets, picnic tables, and dumpsters. Naturally, it requires a Tonto Pass. This parking lot, and the beach, fill up quickly on summer weekends.

GPS Trailhead Coordinates	01 BUTCHER JONES TRAIL: SAGUARO LAKE
UTM zone (WGS 84)	12S
Easting	0452326
Northing	3715004
Latitude/Longitude	
North	33° 34' 31.2"
West	111° 30' 52.1"

SCENERY: ☆ ☆ ☆
TRAIL CONDITION: ☆ ☆
CHILDREN: ☆ ☆ ☆
DIFFICULTY: ☆
SOLITUDE: ☆ ☆

DISTANCE: *8.6 miles*
HIKING TIME: *4 hours 45 minutes*
OUTSTANDING FEATURES: *Views of the lake, desert scenery, fishing access*

Palo Verde Trail 512 is an easy hike around the lake and through the desert, in the event that weather or boredom or crowds have dissuaded you from water activities. In addition to great views of the lake and surrounding countryside, there is a wide variety of desert flora, including a giant, two-headed saguaro, and fields of quartz. You can explore the Sonoran fjords, too. The trail also provides a pedestrian connection between Rattlesnake Cove and SB Cove on the lakeshore.

Palo Verde Trail begins in Rattlesnake Cove on the shining shore of Bartlett Reservoir. In addition to the trailhead, you'll find a couple dozen picnic cabanas, restrooms with flush toilets, paved and marked parking, a campground host, and a water pump. There is also a swimming area several hundred feet down from the cabanas at the lake's usual low level. The cove itself is a "no wake" zone.

Descend the stairs from the restrooms, and you'll notice the trail sign near the manual water pump. After topping off your water containers, head down the path (almost a sidewalk) a couple hundred feet until you reach the true trailhead. To your right, a steep ramp leads down to a fishing pier. A sign to your left explains how that big weird pile of plastic you see on the shore isn't garbage—it's a fish habitat. When you're done sorting out the logic of that, you'll notice the hiker symbol for the trailhead to the immediate right of the fish habitat placard.

Three tracks start from this sign. Do not follow the trail that heads straight down into the wash or the one that marches straight

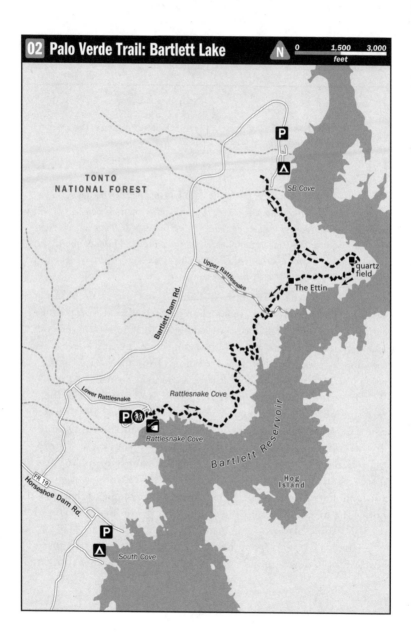

N

0   1,500   3,000
feet

TONTO
NATIONAL FOREST

P

SB Cove

Upper Rattlesnake

quartz
field

The Ettin

Bartlett Dam Rd.

Lower Rattlesnake

Rattlesnake Cove

P

Rattlesnake Cove

Bartlett Reservoir

Hog
Island

FR 19

Horseshoe Dam Rd.

P

South Cove

up the hill. Palo Verde Trail goes between them, along the side of
the hill and around the wash, working its way roughly east, out of the
cove and toward the main body of the lake.

You will cross several washes like this, mostly at or above the
"driftwood line" that marks the highest advance of the lake level. All
of the crossings going out of Rattlesnake Cove work this way.

A fine representation of the lower Sonoran ecosystem sprouts
from the bed of pulverized orange granite that passes for soil around
the lake. Saguaros, palo verde, mesquite and teddy bear cholla are
all common, the latter having an unfortunate tendency to crowd the
trail. This particular sort of cactus has special appeal for nosy dogs,
so if you're hiking with one, keep the leash short.

After three washes, the trail climbs up to about the 1,900-
foot line to wind east, then north, around the hill. Here, you'll
be rewarded with an expansive view of the lake and the mountains
beyond. You can see the Granite Mountains straight across the
way; on a clear day you'll see Four Peaks in the far southeast. To
the northeast, you can see the southern tip of the Mazazatl range.
In good weather, the lake will be crowded with boats, but you'll still
have the trail to yourself.

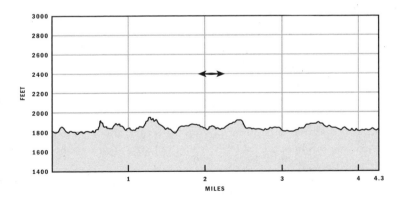

The second wash you cross going north is the first exception to the driftwood rule, going a good deal west, up the shore, to avoid a copse of palo verde trees. Go straight across, and you'll find the fiberglass trail sign. Don't follow the deer trail up the wash.

Over the next ridge, you'll encounter the Sonoran fjords: deep inlets where water juts between steep cliffs. The trail cuts away from the rugged shoreline here to serpentine elaborately up, around, and down various hills. Despite the east-to-west wanderings, you are actually still traveling roughly north. You finally cross a large, sandy wash and encounter the Ettin.

The Ettin is the giant, two-headed saguaro cactus that guards the trail junction. A fiberglass sign near its trunk marks the spot. Here the trail splits: heading westward, up the wash, will take you to SB Cove—a facility much like Rattlesnake Cove; straight ahead, out of the wash, the trail makes it way back toward the shoreline. These trails meet near SB Cove and form a loop. Go up the wash.

The footpath has long washed away. You'll be way-finding from fiberglass post to fiberglass post, and then from rock cairn to rock cairn. If you lose your way, just stay with the wash. As you climb higher, though, the trail begins to emerge, and you'll find yourself on an honest footpath once more. When this trail splits, go west. Follow this path over the hills, and down toward SB Cove.

The spur to SB has been washed out in a few places and is somewhat treacherous. However, unless the lake level is maxed, a dirt road follows the shoreline and proves much easier to traverse.

SB Cove has paved parking, numerous cabanas, and flush toilets, thus providing an excellent mid-hike resting and eating spot. When you are sufficiently refreshed, follow the dirt road back until you feel comfortable hopping back on the trail. A short climb will return you to where the trail splits. You're going to go straight here to finish the loop.

This trail takes you east, then south, around a little peninsula in the lake. Keep an eye out for the quartz field, where numerous chunks of the bright, white mineral litter the hillside—one of the few breaks from the otherwise orange or tan geology. You will also wander through some cool boulder piles, but don't get too distracted because the trail can be faint through here.

The trail turns southward, still staying near the shore, until it cuts a bit inland again and then heads down into the wash, where the Ettin waits patiently for your return.

DIRECTIONS: Follow Cave Creek Road north from Phoenix through the towns of Cave Creek and Carefree. On the far side of Carefree, you will come to the ranger station. Turn right at the station on Horseshoe Dam Road (a.k.a. Forest Road 205). Signs will announce all of this. If you do not have a Tonto Pass, buy one at the ranger station.

Horseshoe Dam Road turns into FR 19. Do not follow the road north; follow the signs east to Bartlett Reservoir. At Bartlett, you'll turn left and follow the signs to Rattlesnake Cove. Rattlesnake Cove requires a Tonto Pass (as does just about everything around Bartlett Lake).

GPS Trailhead Coordinates	02 PALO VERDE TRAIL: BARTLETT LAKE
UTM zone (WGS 84)	12S
Easting	0441638
Northing	3745279
Latitude/Longitude	
North	30° 50' 55.1"
West	111° 37' 58.5"

SCENERY: ⛰ ⛰

TRAIL CONDITION: ⛰ ⛰ ⛰

CHILDREN: ⛰ ⛰ ⛰ ⛰

DIFFICULTY: ⛰

SOLITUDE: ⛰

DISTANCE: *8.6 miles*

HIKING TIME: *5.5 hours*

OUTSTANDING FEATURES: *Cacti, cliffs, city vistas, access to Wind Cave*

This convenient hike is suitable for showing children, dogs, relatives from back East, and other limited hikers the wonders of the desert without many of the hardships of the desert. The trip loops around the slopes of Pass Mountain, in and out of Usery Mountain State Park, in the Goldfield range near Mesa.

🚶 From the trailhead parking, a dirt lot with no services, several trails all wander more or less north and west toward Pass Mountain to the huge wash that separates the trailhead from the slopes like a moat. Large rock cairns mark the trail down into the wash. Look for another cairn about 100 feet "upstream" (roughly north) marking the outbound trail. After emerging from the wash, follow any track about 50 feet upslope to the main trail, which has been pounded white and is as obvious as a sidewalk. Proceed westward up the slope until it turns north to follow along the mountainside.

All of the usual specimens of lower Sonoran vegetation are well represented on this trail: saguaro, ocotillo, and several varieties of barrel, prickly pear, and, of course, cholla cacti.

At 1.6 miles, the trail turns east to begin switchbacking up the orange cliffs. At points the trail has been reduced to bare (and slippery) rock. At the top, where you reach a saddle between Pass Mountain and its immediate neighbor to the east (Peak 3163, named after its elevation), turn around and enjoy the view of all of Apache Junction and most of Mesa. A sharp eye can spot your parked car.

The distinctive cliff line that distinguishes Pass Mountain (and also gave it its other name, Scar Mountain) marks where the

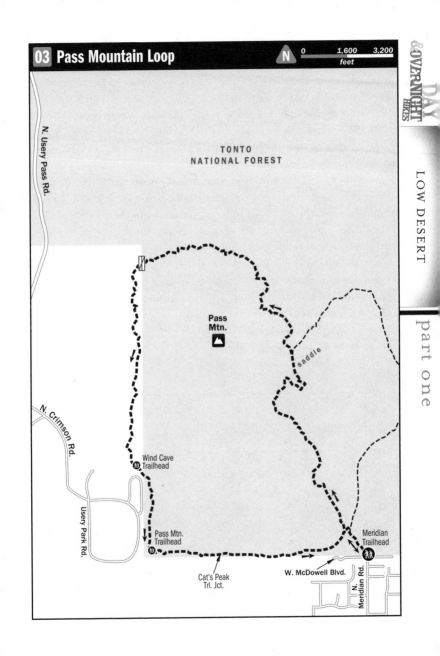

03 Pass Mountain Loop

N   0   1,600   3,200
                      feet

DAY
&OVERNIGHT
HIKES

LOW DESERT

part one

N. Usery Pass Rd.

TONTO
NATIONAL FOREST

Pass
Mtn.

saddle

N. Crimson Rd.

Wind Cave
Trailhead

Usery Park Rd.

Pass Mtn.
Trailhead

Cat's Peak
Trl. Jct.

Meridian
Trailhead

W. McDowell Blvd.

N. Meridian Rd.

granite foundation ends and the cap of volcanic rhyolite begins. This porous rock, aside from being somewhat treacherous to climb, provides an excellent habitat for the bright-yellow lichen that covers the otherwise bright-orange cliffs.

This popular trail has led to many side trails being created by junior high boys; these reflect their level of judgment. The main path is wide and pounded into whiter powder. Stick to it as you go counterclockwise around the slope.

As you round the northern end, you'll encounter the cattle gate that marks the boundary to the state park portion of the hike. At about this point, you'll start to hear gunfire from the gun range that is less than I mile north. Also keep an eye out for the pygmy saguaro and the family of teddy bear cholla cacti.

Winding around the northwest slope, the sound of gunfire fades as you descend into a forest of saguaro cacti. Your halfway mark is the Wind Cave trailhead, about 4.5 miles into your journey. The trailhead has restrooms, a water fountain (!), picnic cabanas, and paved parking. Wind Cave itself, another I.5 miles and about I,000 feet straight up the slope, is unremarkable, being small and frequently overrun with bees.

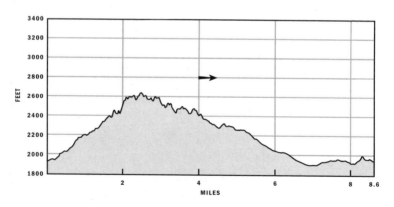

If you know what to look for, the slopes of Pass Mountain are on the front lines of the secret Grass War in the Sonoran Desert. Ranchers and landscapers have, with the best of intentions, introduced grasses to the Sonoran from Africa and warmer parts of the Mediterranean. These exotic grasses share the same drought resistance as their native counterparts and are even similar in appearance.

But you can tell them apart after a fire. Fires are rare in the Sonoran Desert, and the native grasses are not well adapted to it. In contrast, fires are regular events on the African savannahs, and plants native to that area practically depend upon it. Buffelgrass, an African import, both burns readily, even when green, and grows back rapidly after fires—so it starts to crowd out local plants as soon as the smoke clears.

You can find buffelgrass growing alongside native grasses such as fountain grass, big Goleta, and purple three-awn all long the slopes of Pass Mountain—for now.

The state park portion of the trail stays lower on the slope, an even stroll through the desert, tilting only to go in and out of washes. Farther along you'll walk by the Pass Mountain trailhead (also within the state park—fee area) and then past the junction with Cat's Peak Trail, which wanders past that knob of a hill to your right and around the southern reaches of the state park. Soon after that, you will reenter the Tonto.

As you come around the southern slopes, residential neighborhoods creep right up to the forest boundary. People have paid a lot of money to build homes where hikers can look into their backyards. The trail heads due east along this line until it approaches the moat of a wash to complete the loop.

DIRECTIONS: Of the three possible trailheads, Meridian trailhead, at the northern terminus of Meridian Road, is the only one in Tonto National Forest proper and, more importantly, the only one without a fee. The other two lie within the Usery Mountain Recreation Area, a state park that charges $6 a vehicle.

Take the Superstition Freeway (US 60) east into Apache Junction. Exit on Meridian Road and proceed north about 5.5 miles until the road dead-ends at the trailhead.

GPS Trailhead Coordinates	03 Pass Mountain Loop
UTM zone (WGS 84)	12S
Easting	0446080
Northing	3702926
Latitude/Longitude	
North	33° 27' 58.16"
West	111° 34' 48.87"

04 Fish Rock Loop

SCENERY: ✿ ✿ ✿	DISTANCE: *5.5 miles*
TRAIL CONDITION: ✿ ✿	HIKING TIME: *4 hours 50 minutes*
CHILDREN: ✿	OUTSTANDING FEATURES: *Rock formations,*
DIFFICULTY: ✿ ✿ ✿	*cacti, a chance to test your way-finding skills*
SOLITUDE: ✿ ✿ ✿	

This hike, near Mesa, provides some desert solitude without a long drive. The tradeoff, though, is that the trail is steep and hard to follow as you make your way through the relatively pristine desert that surrounds the Goldfield Mountains. After a steep climb up Peak 3163, you cross that saddle that separates it from Bull Dog Ridge and then follow the rock cairns around the backside of this mountain. The return route is a portion of the popular and well-beaten trail around neighboring Pass Mountain.

🚶🚶 Any number of little criss-crossing trails lead roughly north and west from the dirt lot of the Meridian trailhead at the edge of Apache Junction. They all lead to the great moat of a wash that separates the trailhead from the popular Pass Mountain. Along the near side of this wash, though, runs a trail as wide as a road, and traveling north along this path you will find the words "Fish Rock" and an arrow hand painted upon a rock.

Fish Rock is not on any map. The mountain directly north of you (which you will soon be climbing) is officially called Peak 3163; the number refers to its elevation. The name Fish Rock may refer to one or more of the rock formations adorning Bulldog Ridge, which is immediately east of Peak 3163.

Fish Rock Trail follows the wash until it starts to climb the slope of Peak 3163. This climb is steep and rocky but well defined. You'll move a lot of loose rock with your boots. Around the east slope the trail comes to the saddle that separates it from Bulldog Ridge.

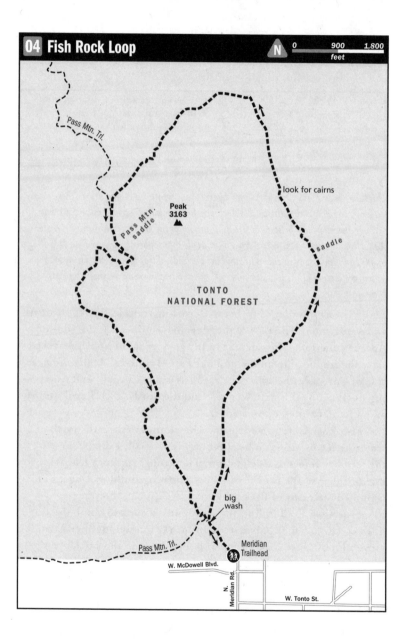

N

0   900   1,800
feet

Pass Mtn. Trl.

Pass Mtn. saddle

Peak 3163 ▲

look for cairns

saddle

TONTO NATIONAL FOREST

big wash

Pass Mtn. Trl.

Meridian Trailhead

W. McDowell Blvd.

N. Meridian Rd.

W. Tonto St.

While you're standing here panting, turn around and gaze at the vista of Apache Junction and most of Mesa, which spreads out before you. To the right of those big green tanks in the foreground lies the tiny parking lot where you left your car. You've gone about 1.4 miles at this point and climbed to 2,600 feet, almost 800 feet above the trailhead.

The trail heading due east across the saddle is a summit trail to the peaks along Bulldog Ridge, which have some cool formations, including a natural arch. But the climb is troublesome, with a thin, steep path choked by cholla cacti. On the left (west) side of the saddle, a narrower trail descends around the mountain. That's your route.

This side of Peak 3163 is a wonderland of cacti: saguaro, barrel, prickly pear, ocotillo, three different species of cholla (buckhorn, cane, and the ubiquitous chain fruit, or jumping, cholla), and small palo verde, all healthy and untrammeled. Birds, rodents, and (depending on the temperature) lizards scurry away, all being genuinely surprised to see humans on this side of the mountain.

However, less than 1 mile past the saddle, the trail becomes

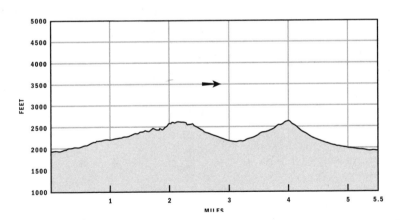

indiscernible, and you must now navigate from rock cairn to rock cairn through the cacti and brush. You'll notice, as you look for piles of rock, the trampoline webs of funnel spiders beneath the various species of cacti. You'll also notice the basalt and other volcanic rocks that speak of the Goldfield's fiery origins.

Should you miss a cairn, the route generally goes upslope of the large wash that circles the north side of Peak 3163. If you find yourself crossing that wash (it's too deep not to notice doing so), you're going too far north. The route eventually winds west then around the peak and uphill toward Pass Mountain.

Halfway up the slope of Pass Mountain, about 3.5 miles into your journey, you should cross Pass Mountain Trail, the popular and obvious route that circumnavigates this ridge. Turn left (south), for this is your route back to the trailhead.

Pass Mountain Trail will cross the saddle that stretches to Peak 3163 and then switchback down to the lower slopes. There is plenty of desert flora along here as well, but you may have been spoiled by the frequency and condition of the specimens on the far side of the peak. What is remarkable are the yellow and orange cliffs that form a band across the Pass Mountain ridgeline. This is where the volcanic rhyolite sits upon the range's hidden granite base. Bright-yellow lichen grows over the top of the bright-orange rhyolite.

After 1.5 miles, the trail will wind to the west around the southern slope, but you will turn off before then—when you see the huge rock cairn. Here, head southeast to cross the big moat of a wash. About 100 feet south of the goat track you took in to the wash, you'll find a goat track out of it. Simply proceed southeast, back to the trailhead.

DIRECTIONS: Take Superstition Freeway (US 60) east into Apache Junction. Exit on Meridian Road and travel north about 5.5 miles until it dead-ends at the trailhead.

GPS Trailhead Coordinates	04 FISH ROCK LOOP
UTM zone (WGS 84)	12S
Easting	0446080
Northing	3702926
Latitude/Longitude	
North	33° 27' 58.16"
West	111° 34' 48.87"

SCENERY: ☆ ☆ ☆	DISTANCE: *15.25 miles*
TRAIL CONDITION: ☆ ☆ ☆ ☆	HIKING TIME: *7 hours*
CHILDREN: ☆ ☆ ☆	OUTSTANDING FEATURES: *Views of Picketpost*
DIFFICULTY: ☆ ☆	*Mountain and other prominences, pristine Sonoran*
SOLITUDE: ☆ ☆ ☆	*Desert, outstanding wildflowers (in season), and a*
	shiny new trail to walk on

This newly renovated trail goes around the convoluted slopes of Picketpost Mountain, climbing up and through Alamo Canyon, and then over and down into Telegraph Canyon. A perfect hike for showing the desert to children and other lesser hikers, without the crowds of more urban hikes, or the need to mount a real expedition. This hike is a part of Arizona Trail (AZT), which runs from Utah to Mexico, and Grand Enchantment Trail, which winds from Phoenix to Albuquerque.

🚶🚶 A tiny memorial sits near the start of the trail in the Picket-post Trailhead. You can sit on one of the rocks that surround a plaque commemorating Wil Passow (1924–1999), AZT blazer and organizer. While many trails were originally laid down for commercial purposes (livestock routes and so forth), almost all of the maintenance and improvement of any trail on public lands is done by volunteers.

Starting east, you cross two washes (actually one big wash with an island in the middle) past signs that warn you not to cross if they're flooded. This portion has been excessively cairned. Follow the packed-dirt singletrack trail through the desert. Prickly pear, hedge-hog, and various cholla cacti pop up around small, almost shrublike mesquite and palo verde trees.

Picketpost Mountain looms ahead of you, and your route will go halfway around its foothills. You soon come to the jeep road that leads to its slopes, but your trail goes straight across, turning southward.

N   0   2,000   4,000
                feet

Arnett Creek

E. Saddleridge Trl.

jeep x-ing

fallen saguaro

TONTO
NATIONAL FOREST

Picketpost
Mtn.

AZT sign

Alamo Canyon Rd.

look north

saguaros

saddle

saguaros

saddle

cholla

Trough
Springs

mesquite

Telegraph Canyon Rd.

DAY
& OVERNIGHT HIKES

LOW DESERT

part one

These foothills are composed of orange volcanic tuff (sprinkled with bright-yellow lichen) covering basalt, covering granite. There is also quartz about, and you start to see barrel cacti. During flower season, you'll see flowers of all colors and sizes, from fragile yellow poppies in late March to flaming cactus flowers in May.

About 1 mile in, notice the big multi-arm saguaro fallen over on the west (right) side of the trail. A quarter mile past this sad landmark, you start climbing up and down the hills. If you pay attention, you'll notice the uphill climbs outnumber the downhill climbs, but none are particularly long or steep.

A multitude of lizards scurry out of your way as you crunch around these hills, especially on a warm day. Wrens dart about among the tops of the stunted trees, while ravens or hawks circle overhead. Primary-colored butterflies flutter about, and in flower season, a host of bees will fill any south-facing slope with an unnerving buzz.

Around the 2-mile mark, the dry wash that defines the bottom of Alamo Canyon will be visible to your right. An intermittent jeep trail runs on the opposite side. The AZT folk carved this trail out as an alternative to that jeep road.

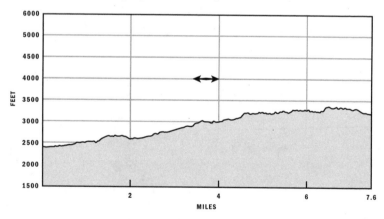

Soon you'll pass by the wash, go over a little bluff, and come down to the wash again. An AZT sign marks this spot, part of an old detour, and most published materials advise following the wash past this point. Don't; follow the trail right in front of you.

The trail starts bending to the east, cutting in and out of a side-wash. You start to see century plants and hackberry bushes, as you cut across the wash several times, until you climb a little to the moldy boulder sitting on the side of the trail, looking like an enormous, rotting bread product. It's not mold, of course, but brown and black lichen.

Immediately past the boulder, you cross through the now weedy wash one last time and then climb uphill a bit to where the trail forks. Stay to the right, the wider trail heading south. You top the hill and cross a grassy little clearing before the trail starts winding south by southeast along the ridgeline.

Stop and turn around: To the left of Picketpost Mountain you can see Weaver's Needle; to the right, Apache Leap.

Continue winding into the upper reaches of Alamo Canyon. Quartz and basalt sparkle beneath your feet. At 5.5 miles, you pass through a stand of saguaros. The trail then switches into and out of a mesquite- and weed-filled wash.

At about the 6-mile mark, you climb out of Alamo Canyon proper to a cholla-crowned saddle separating two tuff-covered hills. That road in the distance, winding along the mountainside, is Telegraph Canyon Road, your eventual destination.

The trail winds south from here, into a tributary of what will eventually become Telegraph Canyon. Go down, around, and back up this drainage to the top of the next hill, heading southeast along the ridge to the next saddle.

The top of that saddle, at 6.5 miles in and about 3,300 feet altitude, is the highest point of the hike. Telegraph Canyon spreads out before you, as the striped hills on the far side rise sharply from the desert floor. You can see a good bit of the trail ahead, winding its way slowly down into the canyon.

Just past 7 miles, you come to an unusually green wash. A cluster of mesquite trees provides some of the only shade you're likely to see on this trail, especially in the middle of the day. In the wash beyond, you find slime- and bug-filled pools fed from Trough Spring. This is a nice place to rest until the bugs find you.

Climb one last little hill from Trough Springs, and you will see the road ahead. Wander another 0.5 miles down through a cluster of chain-fruit cholla and a copse of stunted mesquite trees until you reach the road.

A sign advises hikers to "follow the orange flags to Picketpost trailhead." But you now know that's hardly necessary. Return the way you came.

DIRECTIONS: Take US 60 east from Mesa. Turn off on FR 231 just past Mile Marker 221. Watch out for construction. If you reach Queen Creek Bridge, you've gone too far. Proceed down the graded dirt road and take the signed left turn onto a paved road. This will dead-end in 0.6 miles at the Picketpost Trailhead, which has vaulted toilets but no other facilities. A caretaker works in winter. US 60 is being expanded through here, and these details may change.

	05 ALAMO CANYON TRAIL
GPS Trailhead Coordinates	
UTM zone (WGS 84)	12S
Easting	483542.25
Northing	3681501.66
Latitude/Longitude	
North	N 33° 16' 20.7"
West	W 111° 10' 36.2"

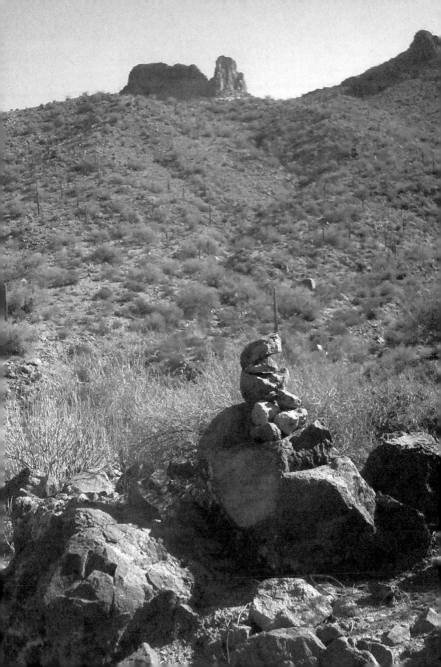

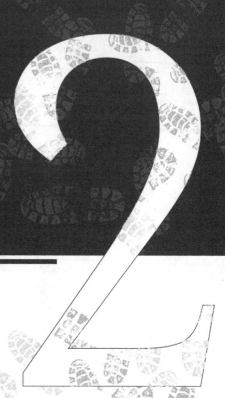

The
Superstition
Wilderness

2

Explore
numerous
high peaks,
deep gorges,
babbling
river
beds,
near-silent
deserts,
hundred-
year-old
mining
camps,
or thousand-
year-old
Native
American
settlements

SCENERY: ✿ ✿ ✿	DISTANCE: *13 miles*
TRAIL CONDITION: ✿ ✿ ✿ ✿	HIKING TIME: *7 hours*
CHILDREN: ✿ ✿	OUTSTANDING FEATURES: *Variable Sonoran*
DIFFICULTY: ✿ ✿ ✿	*vegetation, giant boulders, vistas of mountains,*
SOLITUDE: ✿	*valleys, and the eastern metropolitan area*

From the Broadway trailhead, Jacob's Crosscut Trail follows the slope of the western edge of the Superstition Mountains, with sheer cliffs and giant rock formations on one side, and a panorama of the eastern metropolitan area on the other. The trail leads north to the popular Treasure Loop, a series of short trails that ascend the slopes through big, bizarre rock formations.

🏃🏃 Jacob's Crosscut Trail starts out from the Broadway trailhead near an upscale housing development, but you will climb beyond the backyards after a few minutes. Notice the tall chollas, short palo verde trees, and a good-sized stand of saguaros to your left. To your right, try not to dwell upon the expensive backyards.

A little more than 0.5 miles into the hike, a sign will announce the Gold Mine trail junction. Take the faint trail to the left. This is the only part where the trail may be difficult to locate. As a general rule, where two paths diverge, take the one with the most rocks in it—that is the true trail. It seems as if someone marked the trail by deliberately strewing the path with softball-sized chunks of granite (a.k.a. stumble-rocks—just big enough to turn your ankles unless you keep your attention at your feet). The stumble-rocks come in various shades of pink and red, with lava-black trim. This all leads through a virtual forest of saguaro, palo verde, and tall jumping cholla.

Every time you dare look up from the rock-filled trail, you'll notice the brown cliffs getting steadily closer. Rock cairns will guide

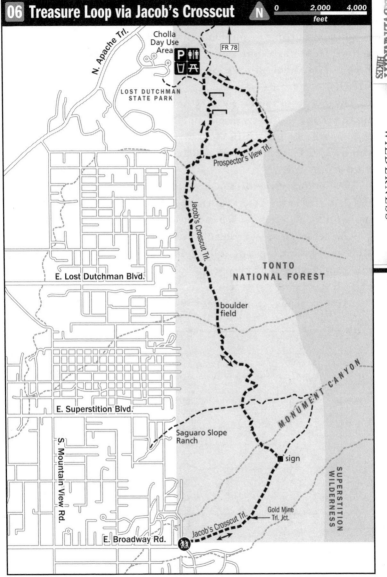

N   0   2,000   4,000
                    feet

Cholla
Day Use
Area

FR 78

LOST DUTCHMAN
STATE PARK

N. Apache Trl.

Prospector's View Trl.

Jacob's Crosscut Trl.

TONTO
NATIONAL FOREST

boulder
field

E. Lost Dutchman Blvd.

E. Superstition Blvd.

S. Mountain View Rd.

Saguaro Slope
Ranch

MONUMENT CANYON

sign

SUPERSTITION
WILDERNESS

Jacob's Crosscut Trl.

Gold Mine
Trl. Jct.

E. Broadway Rd.

you here and there. As long as you are heading uphill and generally northeast, you will be all right.

Soon you come to another sign with the word "Trail" and arrows. Heed it. Past this point, the trail is more obvious and becomes smoother—it's predominantly sand, with only a few rocky stretches.

By this point you are heading north and will continue roughly that direction until Treasure Loop. The trail turns in and out of some sizable ravines. Cliffs loom over you at this point. You'll circumnavigate black and brown boulders, following the slope along the 2,200-foot line.

By the time you cross the second big wash, at just under 3 miles, the character of the desert has changed. You'll notice fewer cacti and more things with leaves, such as brittle brush and acacia bushes.

The desert is an ecosystem of very tight tolerances. The slightest change in drainage and soil conditions can give birth to a whole different regime of plants just 1,000 feet from what seems like an entirely separate ecosystem.

This particular stretch is punctuated with giant boulders. Many

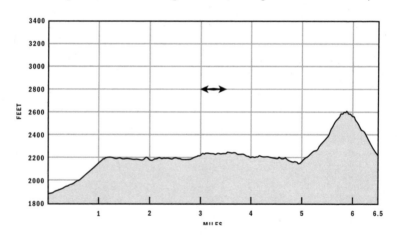

are the size of cars; a few are the size of houses. It's obvious that these chunks of granite were calved from the great cliffs above you and then rolled down to their current perches.

At 4.4 miles, you come to the signed junction with Siphon Draw Trail, which goes up the ravine toward the cliffs. Stay on Jacob's Crosscut. Less than 0.5 miles later, you'll come to the signed junction with Prospector's View Trail. You'll return to this from the other direction. For now, keep going straight.

Here, trail traffic increases: Treasure Loop is one of the most popular trails in the national forest. The trail will wind northeast. Downslope from you lies Lost Dutchman State Park. On a clear day, you can see Four Peaks ahead in the far distance. Cacti start to crowd out leafy plants again. You'll pass a couple of benches along the trail, on either side of a golden, sandy wash. This is about the 5-mile mark.

Soon after the benches, you come to the first (southern) leg of Treasure Loop Trail 56. In good weather, this leg is like a freeway full of day hikers of all ages and abilities. Avoid this particular stretch and keep going straight.

For your information, if you turn left, the trail leads to Cholla Day Use Area, a parking and picnic area, where there are restrooms and a drinking fountain. If you need to, stop in; it's about a 0.5-mile detour down and back. The state park charges a fee for vehicles, but pedestrians coming down from the mountain pay nothing.

Going back up you'll soon intersect the second, northern leg of Treasure Loop. This one is less used, though you'll still likely have a little company. Most people hike up and back via the southern leg.

Jacob's Trail heads north from here, traveling about 1 mile through cholla and palo verde before terminating at Crosscut Trail-head on Forest Road 78. That's a fine stretch of desert and the only part of the trail where civilization is not abundantly evident. But this route goes right, up Treasure Loop.

Treasure Loop is quite wide and heavily trampled, and a fairly steep climb at more than 400 feet in about 1 mile of trudging. There are a couple of benches beside the trail, which charges straight up until near the end then starts to switchback around some large boulders.

Once again, all about you are numerous demonstrations of how gravity and erosion can take huge globs of granite and carve them into abstract art. Turning around, you might notice that in late-afternoon sunlight, the cliffs above you glow, while the Apache Junction and Mesa glitter like a field of broken glass below.

The trail wanders through the wonder rocks, heading south along the 2,600-foot line. Pass the second leg of Treasure Loop to switchback down Prospector's View Trail instead. This route features better vistas and fewer people, and dumps you onto Jacob's Trail closer to your car.

Return south along Jacob's Crosscut to the Broadway trailhead.

DIRECTIONS: Take US 60, Superstition Freeway, east to Apache Junction. Exit on Idaho Road (Exit 196) heading north (left). Less than 2 miles north, you'll take a hard right (northeast) on Old West Highway. Take the next possible left, Broadway Road, heading east. Follow Broadway Road until it ends at a housing development. The trailhead lies at the end of the low wall around a parking lot with room for a mere six cars.

GPS Trailhead Coordinates	06 TREASURE LOOP VIA JACOB'S CROSSCUT
UTM zone (WGS 84)	12S
Easting	0459160
Northing	3697080
Latitude/Longitude	
North	33° 24' 28.6"
West	111° 28' 36.6"

SCENERY: 🌵 🌵 🌵	DISTANCE: *13 miles*
TRAIL CONDITION: 🌵 🌵	HIKING TIME: *7.5 hours*
CHILDREN: 🌵	OUTSTANDING FEATURES: *Cholla forests,*
DIFFICULTY: 🌵 🌵 🌵 🌵 🌵 🌵 🌵	*The Garden, mountain vistas, Battleship Mountain,*
(AFTER HEAVY RAINS)	*all manner of granite formations, and a plain right*
SOLITUDE: 🌵 🌵	*out of a spaghetti western*

This loop ascends from First Water trailhead, climbs through The Garden, then descends through Second Water Canyon to the confluence of Second Water and Boulder creeks. It then follows Boulder Canyon past Battleship Mountain, between Yellow Mountain and the Red Hills, and up into East Boulder Canyon to the junction with Dutchman's Trail. Finally, it follows Dutchman's Trail back to First Water trailhead. The difficulty of this hike is tied to the water level in Boulder Creek.

🚶🚶 Begin on Dutchman's Trail 104 heading roughly southeast. In less than 1 mile, the trail forks at Second Water Trail 236. Go left here, roughly east. Soon after, pick your way across the two creeks (First Water Creek and a tributary) and head up into the hills. The exposed strata of granite form an irregular stairway as you climb.

At the top of the hills lies a forest of cholla of all kinds, including buckhorn, teddy bear, and chain fruit. The fuzzy sorts, teddy bear and chain fruit, are gigantic through here; some are as large as small trees. A little way across this plain, at 1.7 miles in, you'll reach the signed junction with Black Mesa Trail 24. Go straight. Soon after this landmark, you will enter The Garden.

The Garden is a flat, grassy plain with an irregular orchard of stubby trees, mesquite, and palo verde, as well as giant chollas, many of which are taller than the trees. The path through this unique little ecosystem runs straight and flat at the 2,400-foot line, continuing

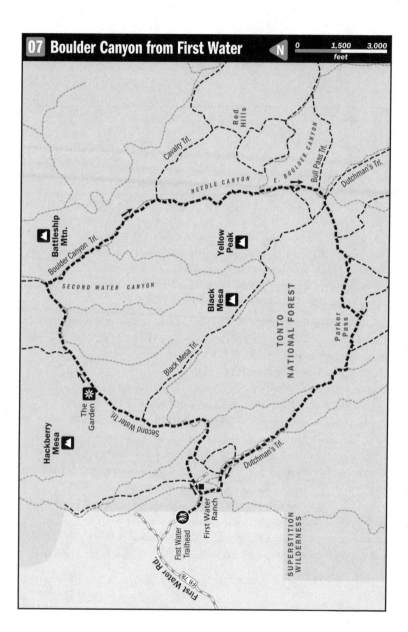

northward about 0.5 miles. At the northern end, you'll find a swimming pool–sized depression, the remains of an old cattle tank.

Past this tank, you're back in the desert. As the trail continues between two hills formed largely of piled lava rock, it becomes the sort of trail that typifies the Superstitions: winding, uneven, crowded with cacti, and chock full of stumble-rocks. Look up to see the sheer-walled, monstrous mesa of Battleship Rock inching closer on the horizon.

The trail winds down into Second Water Canyon. If the water flows, there are some falls in the upper part of the creek. The trail cuts across a ridge and then rejoins the creek below. This lower portion is more riparian, with reeds and mesquite trees.

Second Water Creek empties into Boulder Canyon Creek; their junction is also the trail junction. This signed T-intersection occurs 3.6 miles into the hike. Go right (southeast), where you will immediately cross Boulder Creek. You will do this many, many times as you make your way southeast, up the canyon.

The difficulty of this portion of the hike depends on the water level in Boulder Creek. Most of the time, the creek is dry or close to

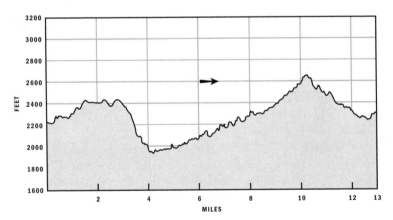

it, making this a moderate hike. After any substantial rain, however, Boulder Creek, as one of the major conduits to Canyon Lake, carries the storm water westward. If Boulder Creek runs strong, the upcoming portion is going to be difficult, and you will soon know precisely how waterproof your footwear is.

Climbing the canyon, you head roughly southeast to pass the looming slopes of Battleship Mountain. Rock cairns occasionally mark the crossings and sometimes lead to an actual trail, though you will find such trails are a bit overgrown, and as much made by water erosion as by foot traffic.

After 1.5 miles of this, the canyon winds more toward the south; around that bend, you'll find the signed junction with Cavalry Trail 239 on the east bank. This trail leads into the Red Hills and points beyond. Stay with Boulder Canyon, which continues to climb south. You see more actual bushes—jojoba and brittlebush—crowding the trail, and fewer cacti, though you will still have to avoid a towering cholla here and there.

Past the Red Hills lies the mouth of Needle Canyon. Shortly past Needle Canyon, you'll come to the confluence of East Boulder Creek and Little Boulder Creek, which form the river (or dry wash) you've been following. Follow the cairns around the left (east) side of the hill that separates the tributaries. This will lead you south to the signed junction with the mighty Dutchman's Trail 104, about 8 miles into the hike. Turn right (south) on Dutchman's.

Less than 1 mile down Dutchman's, you'll find the signed intersection with Black Mesa Trail, which does indeed cross Black Mesa, through a jungle of cholla, to terminate in the intersection you passed on Second Water Trail.

The sign stands in a lonely, flat field with scattered prickly pear and acacia bushes, the kind of place where they leave the hero for dead in spaghetti westerns. The length of that sign's shadow tells you how long you have to get back to your car.

Dutchman's Trail wanders up through jumbled, lichen-covered granite, past the mouths of O'Grady and West Boulder canyons, and then through Parker Pass (stay straight, meaning west). Look for buckhorn cholla, hedgehog cacti, and Engelmann's prickly pear among the palo verde scrubland.

After that rocky climb, the trail descends into First Water Canyon, repeatedly crossing the creek bed. To your left, three striking granite monoliths guard the high slopes of the western edge of the Superstitions. About 3 miles past Parker Pass, you return to the intersection with Second Water Trail. A left turn takes you back the short climb to the trailhead.

DIRECTIONS: Take US 60 east toward Apache Junction. Take Exit 196—Idaho Road—and turn left (north). After 1 mile, turn right (east) on Arizona 88, the Apache Trail. Travel 3.5 miles, following AZ 88 past the Goldfield "ghost town" and Lost Dutchman State Park to reach Forest Road 78. Turn right (east) on FR 78, First Water Road, and follow the graded dirt road for about 3 miles, passing the horse-trailer parking to reach First Water trailhead.

The trailhead has ample (dirt) parking, vaulted toilets, a map, and a registry. Sign in.

GPS Trailhead Coordinates 07 BOULDER CANYON FROM
                           FIRST WATER
UTM zone (WGS 84) 12S
          Easting 0458890
         Northing 3704380
Latitude/Longitude
            North 30° 28' 48.1"
             West 111° 26' 35.2"

SCENERY: ☆ ☆ ☆	DISTANCE: *8.3 miles (plus 1.5-mile side trip)*
TRAIL CONDITION: ☆ ☆ ☆	HIKING TIME: *4.5 hours*
CHILDREN: ☆ ☆	OUTSTANDING FEATURES: *Miner's Needle,*
DIFFICULTY: ☆ ☆ ☆	*several layers of Sonoran vegetation, Bluff Springs,*
SOLITUDE: ☆ ☆	*Crystal Springs, and an army of hoodoos*

This hike follows Dutchman's Trail, the spine of the lower Superstitions, over to Bluff Springs Trail, briefly detouring to the spring itself before continuing down Bluff Springs Trail through some canyons and back to the trailhead.

From the Peralta trailhead, go right at the signed intersection, onto Dutchman's Trail 104. Dutchman's immediately crosses the wash, where the trail forks. Bluff Springs is to the left; Dutchman's is to the right. Go right to start climbing northeast, straight up the hill, through pink and gray tuff covered with all the Sonoran vegetation you'd expect.

To the left, you'll see a fine vista of the Dacite Cliffs, looking like a monstrous sandcastle. To your right, you can see Peralta Road winding through Barkley Basin.

As you round the first hill, now heading northeast, you'll get your first good view of Miner's Needle. Descending the hill, you'll pass an unsigned trail junction. The side trail leads to private ranchland. Stay straight on Dutchman's, making your way northeast across the valley as you traverse a couple of washes.

The Sonoran Desert does well for itself here, sporting cholla, palo verde, saguaro, ocotillo, and brittle bush. The thick vegetation hides all manner of reptiles and rodents, so keep an eye out and be prepared to stop suddenly. Rattlesnakes always have the right of way. Various species of birds circle above as they hunt for reptiles or rodents. Mule deer are often seen in the morning within this basin.

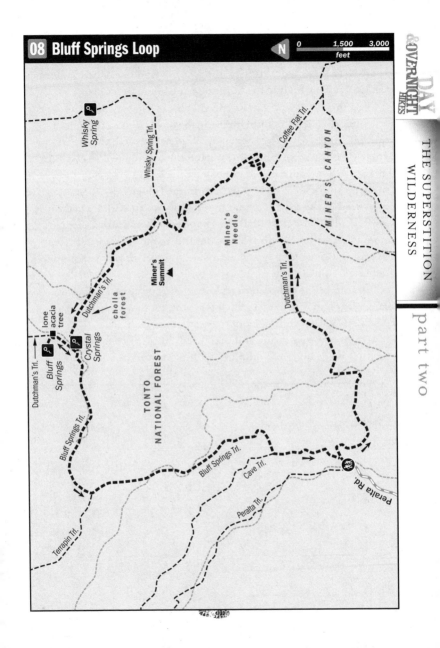

08 Bluff Springs Loop

N

0   1,500   3,000
feet

Whisky Spring

Whisky Spring Trl.

Coffee Flat Trl.

MINER'S CANYON

Miner's Needle

Miner's Summit ▲

cholla forest

Dutchman's Trl.

Dutchman's Trl.

lone acacia tree

Dutchman's Trl.

Bluff Springs

Crystal Springs

TONTO NATIONAL FOREST

Bluff Springs Trl.

Bluff Springs Trl.

Cave Trl.

Peralta Trl.

Terrapin Trl.

Peralta Rd.

The trail bends east at about the 2-mile mark to climb the southern slope of the hill that hosts Miner's Needle and several other outcrops. Near the top of this first climb, you'll find the signed junction with Coffee Flat Trail 108. Continue straight on Dutchman's.

Past this junction, a series of switchbacks leads up, around, and ultimately through the hills, after which your trail turns north. To your left, you can see the (normally) blue sky through the eye of Miner's Needle across the canyon from the hillside you're climbing. This hole in the outcrop is not geologically impressive, but it is a landmark in the Lost Dutchman Goldmine "clues."

Ahead in the distance you can see a big, weird rock formation—a vertical pile of boulders called a "hoodoo." Don't take a picture yet, as the trail goes up to and around this rock. As you wind closer, the trail will cross long stretches of bare rock on an easy but slippery grade.

On top of the saddle next to Miner's Summit, you'll find the signed junction with Whisky Spring Trail 238. Stay straight on Dutchman's. Descending from the saddle, the trail makes a big U around the top of a ravine and then heads northwest. Directly ahead, you'll see the yellow cliffs of Bluff Springs Mountain.

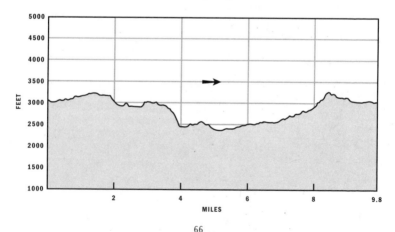

The packed-dirt trail meanders across the flat valley lined with yucca and century plants, pancake prickly pear, an occasional juniper tree, and tall prairie grass. When you're almost across the valley, you'll pass a surreal little forest of cholla. Shortly after the cholla copse, you'll approach Bluff Springs Mountain. Cross the wash to find the junction with Bluff Springs Trail 235, which is surrounded by sugar sumac trees. Any water in that wash, often in algae-lined pools, comes from Crystal Springs.

Continue north on Dutchman's for a little side trip to Bluff Springs itself. Dutchman's Trail opens up into a dusty track across a desert plain. Soon, you'll encounter a lone acacia tree. Look for rock cairns to your left. (If you pass the tree, you've missed them.) The cairns indicate little more than a thin trail. You still have to push through some brush to find Bluff Springs, which is nothing more than a pipe dripping into a bowl of rocks.

Returning to the junction, go west on Bluff Springs Trail, following the wash up toward a little saddle. The trail cuts in, across, and out of the wash several times. Down past that saddle, you'll come to the signed junction with Terrapin Trail 234. Continue straight as the path now heads south on Bluff Springs. Climb the hill to exit the wash and follow the ridgeline while the drainage itself falls precipitously to your right. Your route ascends the ridge, passing three distinct hoodoos, and then begins a knee-jarring descent, winding its way through tank-sized boulders down into Barks Canyon. The wash and the trail are the same through much of the canyon. The trail will climb out to head south before the canyon itself bends sharply east.

Continue roughly south down, around, and then back up the ridgeline. If you dare look up from the rock-strewn trail, you can see Miner's Needle to your left, along with the whole diorama of the eastern Superstition Wilderness. As you go over the top of the last hill, the trail proper does indeed cut through the rocky summit to turn back and start its descent. At that spot, though, there will be an almost equally prominent side trail heading east. Watch for this, and make sure you take the path that cuts across the top. From that point, Bluff Springs Trail winds steeply and steadily back toward the trailhead.

DIRECTIONS: From Apache Junction, take US 60 east about 8.5 miles to the Peralta Road turnoff. There is a residential development here, but past that cluster of new homes, the road becomes the graded dirt track of Forest Road 77, which, in about 8 miles, will dead-end at the Peralta trailhead. The trailhead has dirt parking, vault toilets, a posted map, a trail log to sign, and, in season, there is often a ranger nearby. It does not have trashcans or water.

GPS Trailhead Coordinates	08 BLUFF SPRINGS LOOP
UTM zone (WGS 84)	12S
Easting	467648.13
Northing	3695418.54
Latitude/Longitude	
North	33° 23' 51.3"
West	111° 20' 52.4"

SCENERY: 🌂 🌂 🌂	SOLITUDE: 🌂
TRAIL CONDITION: 🌂 🌂 🌂 /🌂	DISTANCE: *4.6 miles*
CHILDREN: 🌂 🌂 🌂 /🌂	HIKING TIME: *3.5 hours*
(PERALTA/CAVE)	OUTSTANDING FEATURES: *Weaver's Needle,*
DIFFICULTY: 🌂 🌂 🌂	*cool rock formations, view of the western Superstitions*

Peralta Trail up to Fremont Saddle is, despite its difficulty, one of the most popular hikes in the Superstitions for a reason. Everything you're likely to find in the western Superstitions is piled around this steep route and, at the end, you encounter a jaw-dropping vista of Weaver's Needle, the signature rock formation of this mountain range. The hike then follows a faint side track to a remote but even better view of the Needle; follow cairns and your intuition along Cave Trail, down to its junction with Bluff Springs Trail, which leads back to the trailhead.

🚶🚶 From the Peralta trailhead, take the left at the signed intersection, up Peralta Trail 102. The name Peralta comes from the legendary, if not strictly historical, 1850s Mexican mining expedition that ran afoul of Apache (or possibly Yavapai) warriors and was slain to the man.

The trail starts north and starts climbing—get used to that. To your left, the Dacite cliffs tower above you like some monstrous, deformed pipe organ. The trail bends northwest after 0.25 miles, climbing up the steep-walled canyon. You're in for a stairway-grade climb, all the way up. Level stretches are the exception as you wander up, around, and through ochre boulders and a wide variety of brush. You pass through some open desert when you climb the slopes away from the ravine, but then you cross the ravine again, through more brush.

This stretch of the trail is the most heavily used route in the wilderness area proper; in fact, it's one of the most heavily used

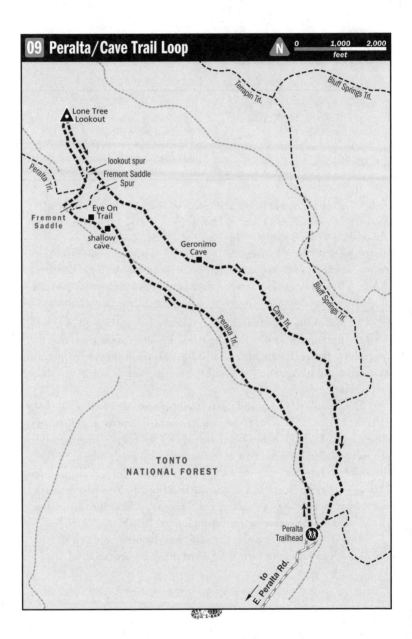

09 Peralta/Cave Trail Loop

N

0   1,000   2,000

feet

Terrapin Trl.

Bluff Springs Trl.

Lone Tree Lookout

Peralta Trl.

lookout spur

Fremont Saddle Spur

Fremont Saddle

Eye On Trail

shallow cave

Geronimo Cave

Bluff Springs Trl.

Cave Trl.

Peralta Trl.

TONTO NATIONAL FOREST

Peralta Trailhead

to E. Peralta Rd.

wilderness trails in the United States. On a weekend with good weather, you'll have a lot of company.

Near the top of the canyon, at about 1.75 miles, you come to a shallow cave. The trail winds around and over the orange rock the cave burrows into. Brick-colored lava rock lies scattered about, as the route straightens and climbs toward Eye On the Trail, a hole-in-rock formation. Fremont Saddle lies just beyond this formation.

At the windswept saddle, you encounter the postcard-quality view of Weaver's Needle that draws so many to this spot. You've climbed more than 1,300 feet in just over 2 miles to get to this point, so take some time to enjoy the view. Weaver's Needle, named for the legendary scout Pauline Weaver, bolts 1,200 feet straight up from the floor of Boulder Canyon to a top elevation of 4,553 feet and is visible from all over the region.

Near the north side of the saddle—and you'll have to hunt for it—is the unsigned spur that leads to Cave Trail. Alternately, you could continue on the Peralta just past the saddle. The path winds north, but just before it cuts back sharply south again to begin its descent into Boulder Canyon, you'll see a cairned side trail climbing

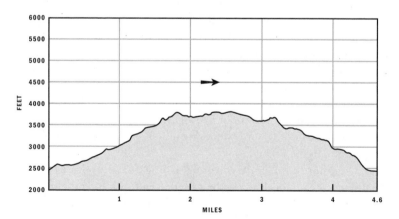

along the side of the ridge. At the far north end of the ridge, you can see a lone pine tree—that's your destination.

This side trail is unofficial, barely more than a game trail where it leaves the main track. There are two ways to go, depending on which set of cairns you end up following. The low route goes around the western edge of the bluff, sometimes getting uncomfortably close to the brink. You'll have to pick your way through the ankle-high maze of lava rock and hedgehog cacti that cover the ridgetop. The high road is less exciting but more straightforward, following the top of the ridge-line. Both routes deteriorate to require you to clamber over boulders and through brush just before you reach the lookout itself.

The lookout is worth finding, if you don't mind a little scram-bling. Besides a stunning view of the Needle, you'll find the place very peaceful. When you have achieved harmony, head back east across the ridgetop, following the Cave Trail.

Cave Trail has no signs. You'll have to follow the cairns across the ridgeline through a wonderland of rock formations. If you're not comfortable with that, or if you are in any danger of running out of daylight, your surest bet is to return down Peralta Trail. Go straight (roughly southeast) past the intersection with the Fremont Saddle spur trail, roughly marked with a line of rocks. Century plants and ocotillo dot this sky island. Cool rock formations jut up all around, accompanied by a 360-degree panoramic view of the Superstitions.

About halfway along the route (about 1.25 miles past Fremont Saddle), and just south of the highest point on the ridge, you pass Geronimo Cave, which has no known association with the legend-ary Apache shaman (who is not known even to have set foot in the Superstitions); this is not really a cave either—just a wide but shallow depression in the rock.

Continue to follow the cairns or, failing that, the obvious route across the ridgeline. As the path descends, winding slightly southward, remember to stay on top of the ridgeline. Stay out of the ravines on either side, unless you are up for some truly brutal bushwhacking. The route dumps you into a little saddle, where it makes an unsigned junction with Bluff Springs Trail 235. After you've picked your way across the ridge, Bluff Springs Trail will seem blazingly obvious. Follow it right (south) as it steeply descends back toward the trailhead.

DIRECTIONS: From Apache Junction, take US 60 east about 8.5 miles to the Peralta Road turnoff. There is a residential development here, but past that cluster of new homes, the road becomes the graded dirt track of Forest Road 77, which, in about 8 miles, will dead-end at the Peralta trailhead. The trailhead has dirt parking, vault toilets, a posted map, and a trail log to sign; in season, there is often a ranger nearby. It does not have trashcans or water.

GPS Trailhead Coordinates	09 PERALTA/CAVE TRAIL LOOP
UTM zone (WGS 84)	12S
Easting	467648.13
Northing	3695418.54
Latitude/Longitude	
North	33° 23' 51.3"
West	111° 20' 52.4"

SCENERY: ☆ ☆ ☆	DISTANCE: *4.3 miles*
TRAIL CONDITION: ☆ ☆ ☆	HIKING TIME: *2 hours*
CHILDREN: ☆ ☆ ☆ ☆	OUTSTANDING FEATURES: *Riparian glades,*
DIFFICULTY: ☆	*isolated meadow, wildlife, a confluence of canyons*
SOLITUDE: ☆ ☆ ☆	*and trails, cowboy ruins*

This hike goes up along Pinto Creek and into a convergence of canyons and trails called Oak Flat (not to be confused with the campground near Superior). As one of the few hikes in this area that does not require expeditionary resources, it is perfect for a day hike or a super-easy overnight. So, feel free to bring the kids and dogs. Both the trailhead and Oak Flats have cowboy ruins to explore; there is also access to a multitude of side trails.

🚶🚶 Take West Pinto Trail 212 from Miles trailhead. These are the remains of Miles Ranch, also called Kennedy Ranch. The Forest Service purchased the wilderness portion in 1986, and the rest of the ranch in 1997, though portions are still used for livestock grazing.

After passing through some oak and juniper, you come to a small field that has eroded down to bare dirt—a possible testament to the effects of grazing. To your right is a fenced pasture. Cross the dirt slope and follow the fence through a marked wilderness-boundary gate and past a long established, though dusty, campsite to reach the intersection with Bull Basin Trail. This path lies near the confluence of the West Fork of Pinto Creek, which runs east—west through here, and Rock Creek, which drains into the Pinto from the southwest.

Bull Basin heads up Rock Creek going south, but stay on Pinto Trail as it crosses and then follows the Pinto wash, heading west through the juniper and oak woodlands. Poison ivy grows near the river, as does manzanita and live scrub oak, but the ivy is the plant you definitely want to watch for.

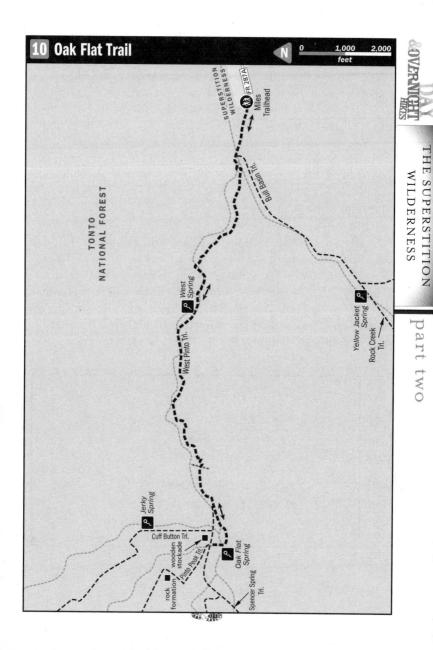

In less than 1 mile, the river bends sharply to pass between two low cliffs. Here the trail and the streambed run the same narrow course through the cliffs. You cross the stream twice, dancing on top of the rocks, for there is no dirt path and there are few cairns to guide you. Once through this passage, though, the trail on either side is relatively obvious.

You then climb, steeply, up and down two bluffs as you climb the canyon into the mountains. You'll pass an old fence as you cross the second bluff. Beyond these bluffs, around the 2-mile mark, the canyon opens up a bit into a wide, level basin where four drainages and four trails converge at Oak Flats.

Pass the signed intersection with Cuff Button Trail, which provides access to several springs up the slopes to the northeast. The climb out of Oak Flats is steep and overgrown, but the rest of the trail is easy to moderate. Stay on Pinto, though. Just past this, cross a clearing covered only with manzanita bushes and sand, and pass the junction with Spencer Spring Trail. That route follows Spencer Canyon, carving out the bottom of Sawtooth Ridge. Numerous floods have left the trail steep and difficult to follow. Stay on Pinto and cross the creek.

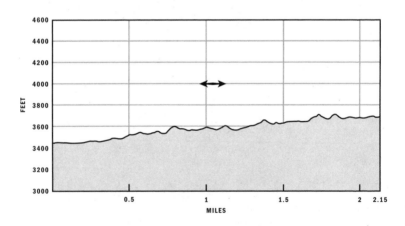

The rocks beneath Pinto Creek turn from brick-orange to blood-red beneath the water, which only complements these mountains' spooky theme. This whole canyon area, bounded by the Sawtooth Ridge to the south and the East Superstition Divide to the north, supports deer, bighorn sheep, and even elk, along with the usual cast of lizards, rodents, and snakes.

Across the creek is the large, oak-lined meadow. Nearby is a circular stockade, which remains as a testament to the strength of bailing wire and cowboy engineering. Other remnants of cowboy living—cabin foundations and the like—can be found among the oaks, manzanita, and bear grass, but it takes some looking.

The Flats provides an excellent selection of camping and picnicking spots. If you want a better view, Pinto, Campaign, and Cuff Button all climb quickly and steeply out of the basin. The best path is Campaign: the grade might be soul crushing, but the trail is unobstructed by brush, and it leads, in less than 1 mile, to chocolate-covered rock formations. When you reach these, turn around to see the whole Flats spread out before you. Return the way you came.

DIRECTIONS: From Apache Junction, take US 60 east 44 miles past Superior and a small community called "Top-o-the-World." Turn left on Pinto Valley Road (FR 287) between mileposts 239 and 240. Pinto Valley Road is a partially paved maze through giant mining operations. Mining companies' penchant for moving whole hills around makes maps useless, but they have put up many signs stating which road is public and which roads definitely are not. Take your time, pay attention, and you should find your way through.

Follow this route about 6.5 miles to FR 287A, an intersection marked by a large sycamore tree and a car-camping area. This dirt road has a reasonable grade but many rocks and ruts. You need a medium-clearance or higher vehicle past this point. Turn left, and wind 5.5 miles up into the canyons on this road, bearing in mind that it will seem longer. The road dead-ends at Miles trailhead, on the site of an old ranch. Near the parking area, a cattle pen and a small shed still stand. Large sycamore and oak trees shade the lot, providing an excellent area for car camping. However, there are no services here.

GPS Trailhead Coordinates	10 OAK FLAT TRAIL
UTM zone (WGS 84)	12S
Easting	493718
Northing	3699801
Latitude/Longitude	
North	33° 26' 15.3"
West	111° 04' 03.3"

SCENERY: ☆ ☆ ☆	DISTANCE: *11.2 miles*
TRAIL CONDITION: ☆ ☆ ☆	HIKING TIME: *8.5 hours*
CHILDREN: ☆ ☆ ☆	OUTSTANDING FEATURES: *Riparian glades and*
DIFFICULTY: ☆ ☆	*woodlands, native American cliff dwellings, cool rock*
SOLITUDE: ☆ ☆ ☆	*formations, caves, a wide meadow where trails and*
	canyons converge

This hike follows the streambed down into Rogers Trough, passing by and around all manner of trees and boulders. Toward the end, you can explore the 600-year-old cliff dwellings up the canyon slope, then Angel Basin itself, a meadow opening up where three canyons converge. This can be done as a long but undemanding day hike or as an easy overnight. The estimated hiking time includes exploring the ruins and riverbeds (and taking the uphill return).

🚶‍♀️🚶 From Rogers Trough trailhead, take Reavis Ranch Trail 109, heading roughly north through the catclaw-dotted pastures. This is part of an active grazing allotment, and you may encounter cows. Because cattle graze upstream, none of the water flowing through the canyon is potable. Sorry.

You'll soon pass the junction with West Pinto Creek Trail, which climbs east over Iron Mountain (that red peak to your right) and into Pinto Creek Canyon. Keep going straight (north) along Reavis Ranch Trail. This route is part of the Arizona Trail (which runs from Mexico to Utah), at least for a while. The singletrack follows the streambed across the chaparral. The farther you go, though, the more oaks start to shade the way.

At 1.5 miles, you come to the intersection with Rogers Trough Trail 110. Reavis Trail heads northeast, up Grave Canyon, toward Reavis Ranch, but your route descends northwest into Rogers Trough. Take the left. Rogers Trough passes through a manzanita

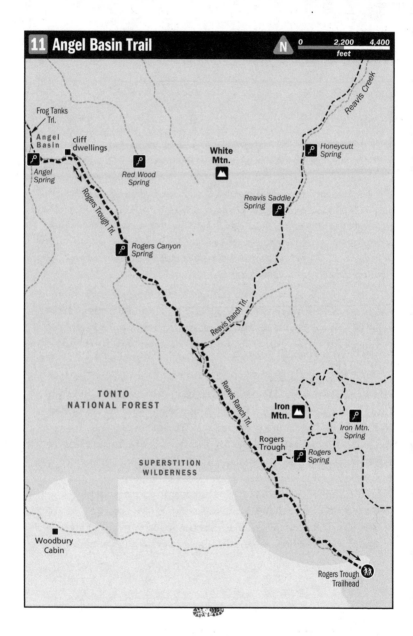

N

0   2,200   4,400
feet

Frog Tanks
Trl.

Angel
Basin

cliff
dwellings

Angel
Spring

Red Wood
Spring

White
Mtn.

Honeycutt
Spring

Reavis Creek

Reavis Saddle
Spring

Rogers Trough Trl.

Rogers Canyon
Spring

Reavis Ranch Trl.

TONTO
NATIONAL FOREST

Reavis Ranch Trl.

Iron
Mtn.

Iron Mtn.
Spring

SUPERSTITION
WILDERNESS

Rogers
Trough

Rogers
Spring

Woodbury
Cabin

Rogers Trough
Trailhead

thicket and across the stream. Continue to follow the right (east) bank of this Arizona sycamore–lined creek through alternating thickets of manzanita and/or catclaw, crossing the stream several times.

In general, the trail becomes more twisted and rockier as it goes deeper into the canyon, which can be great fun if you are in the habit of watching your step. Sometimes it wanders through the shade of tall oak trees; sometimes it meanders through a dusty field of catclaws. Regardless, it always makes its way back to the creek.

At about 11 miles, alligator juniper joins the oak and sycamore in the creekside forest. Birds flutter through all of them as lizards run amok on the rocks. The canyon walls start to close in, and if the trees aren't shading you, the towering hills crowned with orange monoliths that form the canyon will block the morning or late-afternoon sun.

At 11.2 miles, you face a tricky rock-scramble of a river crossing. Past this, follow the now obvious singletrack up and over the bluff through big oak, big Arizona sycamores, and big granite boulders. The river will bend west, and that's when you need to keep an eye out for the caves on the cliffs to your right. Within one of those caves is the Rogers Canyon Cliff Dwelling. You'll have to cross the river to

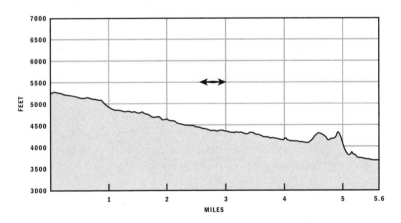

find the steep and unofficial spur trail leading up the slope to the site. Here, the Salado people used loose stone and adobe to wall in a couple of shallow caves. A Forest Service sign gives some history and warns you that it is illegal to disturb the site.

The Salado people are related to the Hohokam, whose adobe ruins and ingenious canals covered much of what is now the Phoenix area. The whole civilization disappeared, however, around 1450 AD—from drought, political strife, or both. The Salado formed a small, and presumably more isolated, portion of that much larger culture.

A wall completely covers the first cave's mouth, but you can walk into a second cave without disturbing the fragile architecture. Black moss covers the stone in the rear of the shallow cave. These ruins are not extensive, having only a couple of rooms, but they are in relatively good shape. Turn around for some insight into why they built this structure here: the view up the canyon is spectacular.

A half mile past the ruins, the canyon opens up into Angel Basin. Here you find the junction with Frog Tanks Trail within a wide meadow with established campsites separated by a maze of catclaws. Oaks, sycamore, and Arizona walnut line the streambeds where three drainages converge. The up-slope edges of the clearing are lined with scrub juniper and netleaf hackberry.

Both Frog Tanks Trail and the rest of Rogers Trough Trail provide more riparian playgrounds to explore, but the hike proper ends at Angel Basin. When you have satisfied your curiosity, return the way you came.

Camping: Angel Basin is popular with campers, mosquitoes, and ants. If that sounds too crowded, you can push up north along Frog Tanks Trail to more-isolated campsites (though the skeeters will doubtless still keep you company). If you do so, keep an eye out for some amazingly large yucca plants growing near the stream.

DIRECTIONS: From Apache Junction, take US 60 east 2 miles past Florence Junction. Make a left at the Queen Valley Road turnoff. After 2 paved miles, follow Hewitt Station Road, which branches to the right, turning to gravel. After about 3 miles, turn left on JF Road (FR 172). Follow this road 8 miles to reach the intersection with Rogers Trough Road (FR 172A). Follow this very rough road 3 miles to the trailhead.

Note that you can probably get to the start of 172A with a high-clearance vehicle, but the last 3 miles require a 4WD. Also note that these roads cross Queen Creek several times, and it is impassable if flooded.

GPS Trailhead Coordinates	11 ANGEL BASIN TRAIL
UTM zone (WGS 84)	12S
Easting	485023.8
Northing	3696115
Latitude/Longitude	
North	33° 24' 15.3"
West	111° 09' 39.8"

SCENERY: ☘ ☘ ☘ ☘	DISTANCE: *34.15 miles*
TRAIL CONDITION: ☘ ☘	HIKING TIME: *23 hours (3 days)*
CHILDREN: ☘	OUTSTANDING FEATURES: *Spectacular*
DIFFICULTY: ☘ ☘ ☘ ☘	*vistas, wildlife, isolation, two historic ranch sites,*
SOLITUDE: ☘ ☘ ☘ ☘	*two Native American ruins, all manner of cool rock*
	formations

This route follows or touches upon all the major routes in the eastern Superstition Wilderness. Climbing up Pinto Creek, the trail crosses over Iron Mountain, descends through Rogers Trough, and passes some 600-year-old cliff dwellings before reaching Angel Basin. The second leg climbs up Paradise Canyon and across Plow Saddle, then winds down past historic Reavis Ranch and Circlestone sites to descend into the pine-forested canyon of Campaign Creek. The third (and easiest) leg follows Campaign Creek up the canyon, past Pinto Mountain, and then down to Oak Flats, to reunite with Pinto Creek. The average elevation gain is more than 1,000 feet per day. This may be the most challenging hike in the book.

🏃 From Miles trailhead, head west on West Pinto Trail 212, which follows the southern edge of the old ranch pasture through juniper and oak woodlands. You quickly cross the wilderness boundary, and then pass the intersection with Bull Basin Trail, immediately after which you cross the wash. About 1 mile in, you cross the wash a couple more times; keep an eye out for poison ivy. Although you climb a couple of steep bluffs, poison ivy represents the only real hazard on the early portion of this trail.

At just past 2 miles, there is an open area called Oak Flats, where several creeks and trails merge. Pass the signed intersections of Cuff Button Trail, Spencer Spring Trail, and Campaign Trail, being sure to stay on West Pinto Trail, following the west fork of Pinto Creek up the canyon. The water level in Pinto Creek through here is a good indicator

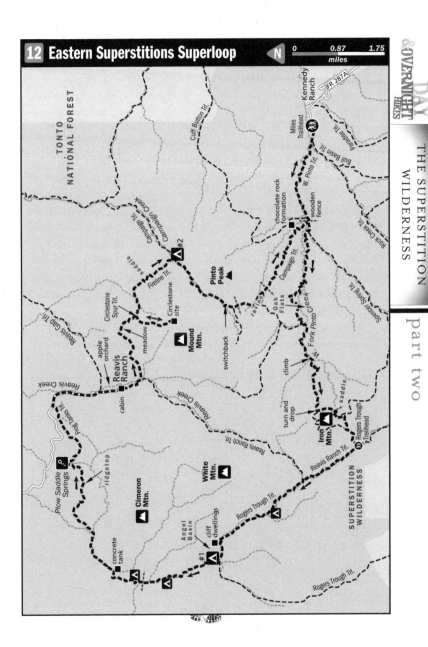

12 Eastern Superstitions Superloop

N

0   0.87   1.75
miles

TONTO
NATIONAL FOREST

Cuff Button Trl.

Campaign Creek

Campaign Trl.

saddle

Fireline Trl.

#2

Pinto Peak

Circlestone Spur Trl.

Circlestone site

Reavis Gap Trl.

apple orchard

meadow

Mound Mtn.

Reavis Ranch

cabin

switchback

ravine

chocolate rock formation

wooden fence

Miles Trailhead

Kennedy Ranch

FR 287A

W. Pinto Trl.

Bull Basin Trl.

Paradise Trl.

Rock Creek Trl.

Spencer Spring Trl.

Oak Flats

W. Fork Pinto Creek

climb

Reavis Creek

Reavis Creek

Reavis Ranch Trl.

Frog Tanks Trl.

Plow Saddle Springs

ridgetop

Cimeron Mtn.

White Mtn.

Angel Basin

cliff dwellings

#1

concrete tank

turn and drop

Iron Mtn.

saddle

Rogers Trough Trailhead

Reavis Ranch Trl.

Rogers Trough Trl.

SUPERSTITION
WILDERNESS

Rogers Trough Trl.

of your water situation for the whole hike. If the stream is flowing, you may be drying your boots by the campfire every night. If it is dry, you are in for a tense scramble between a series of unreliable springs.

Soon the trail climbs a bluff. If you're lucky, the creek babbles a couple hundred feet below. The stones lining the bottom of Pinto Creek turn brick-red, making the water look like a river of blood from the top of the bluff.

At the 3.5-mile mark, you reunite with the creek and follow it closely for another mile. At the 4.5-mile mark, at the 4,200-foot line, you start climbing another bluff. The path is much more overgrown here, with manzanita and scrub oak joining catclaw to block the way.

After a few hundred feet, though, you reach a break in the bushes. The trail becomes easier, with overgrowth the exception to the tall grass that otherwise lines the sparkling basalt pathway. At this point, you should take some time to assess how anything on the outside of your pack has fared, because this was just a training exercise for the real climb to come.

Just past 6 miles, the trail pulls away from the creek for good and you start toward the divide. The grade is steeper, the gravel looser,

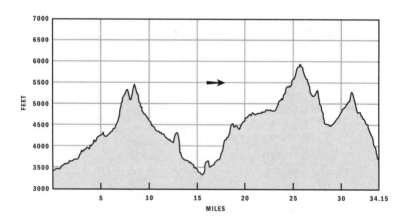

and the overgrowth thicker as you fight your way up the ridge toward Iron Mountain (the one with the big, red rock formation on top).

Toward the top of this ridge, the manzanita separates a bit to provide a straight, though seriously steep, passageway. While relatively clear, the grade is relentless all the way to the 7.2-mile mark, where the trail suddenly turns south and starts dropping. Keep an eye out for hawks, known to nest nearby, as you pick your way across the juniper-lined eastern slope of Iron Mountain. You soon pass a fence, at the 5,000-foot line, and that marks the start of the final series of switchbacks toward the saddle south of the peak.

At 8.2 miles, and 5,470 feet, you reach the top of the saddle—which means you've climbed more than 1,000 feet in 2.2 miles, against a determined defense. Past the saddle, start switchbacking down the mountainside, heading south by southwest, following the wash for a bit. After that, you'll follow the ridgeline a bit. Toward the bottom, cross a shady wash near Rogers Spring. Shortly thereafter, at about 8.9 miles, the trail follows a pipeline, which means you're almost to the bottom. You leave the pipeline and go through a fence to cross a little prairie of high grass and catclaw to reach the junction with Reavis Ranch 109.

Rogers Trough trailhead, a dirt lot with no services, is within sight to the left. Go right (roughly northwest). The rocky little singletrack marches through relatively open terrain along the creek. About a half mile down, oaks start to shade your way as you head down into Rogers Canyon, crossing the creek a couple times as you do so. The terrain becomes more wooded and riparian, with Arizona sycamores and walnut, Fremont cottonwood, and various oak and pine trees all shading the canyon. The farther down you go, the stronger the creek flows. White Mountain looms in the distance ahead.

At 10.7 miles, you leave the Reavis to go left (northwest) on Rogers Trough Trail 110. This route follows the creek closely down the canyon, winding around oaks and boulders, and crossing the water several times.

As you near Angel Basin, keep an eye on the rocky slopes to your right. Within one of those caves is the Rogers Canyon Cliff Dwelling. You'll have to cross the river to find the steep and unofficial spur trail leading upslope to the shallow caves, with entrances partially or completely blocked by the loose-stone construction made by the Salado 600 years ago. These ruins are not extensive; there are only a couple of rooms, but they are in relatively good shape. A Forest Service sign gives some history and warns you that it is illegal to disturb the site.

A half mile past the ruins, you arrive at the junction with Frog Tanks Trail, in a confluence of canyons known as Angel Basin. Several campsites dot the wide meadow, each separated by a maze of catclaw, scrub juniper, and netleaf hackberry.

Angel Basin is popular with campers, mosquitoes, and ants. At night, hundreds of bats emerge from the nearby caves to feast upon the mosquitoes that have been feasting upon the campers. As the night goes on, you may discover that all the cold air in the Superstitions tends to collect in the basin, producing a temperature drop of 40°F or more from the afternoon high. Layer up.

On day two, follow Frog Tanks Trail 112 singletrack north (right at the junction) through the riparian woodland. This section sees less use than Rogers Trough Trail, making it a little more overgrown and occasionally treacherous. You circumnavigate boulder fields and scramble over fallen trees, but it is easy enough to follow, unless you are crossing the river. Many trail signs have been washed away; keep a sharp eye for cairns and use good judgment, or you could be whacking through brush and boulders for quite some time.

Just past 14 miles, near the confluence with Rough Canyon up to the east, and Fish Creek Canyon down west, you pass through a barbed-wire fence. Go straight (north) across the wash, and then across Fish Creek into the juniper stand beyond. Now you cut away from the river, turning northeast on what will become a switchback route up the ridgeline. Shortly, you will climb out of the trees and into transition desert dominated by prickly pear, agave, and cane cholla. Prickly pear pads mix with the clinking basalt stumble-rocks to add extra hazards if you don't step carefully. When you stop to pant, gaze across the three canyons for a 270-degree view of fantastic, chocolate-colored rock formations: pillars, hoodoos, and cliffs of every weird variety.

The trail levels out along the 3,600-foot line to pick its way north across the prickly pear garden near the ridgetop. By the 15.9-mile mark, you're heading steeply downhill over loose basalt rocks of all sizes and along the fence that separates you from a 200-foot drop into a side ravine.

By the 16-mile mark, at which point you've descended 200 feet, the trail levels out into a packed-earth singletrack through mesquite and juniper scrub country. Soon, you pass a concrete cattle tank; it's usually dry, but you can hear Willow Creek below you as you begin your march into Paradise Canyon.

The track stays mostly on the south bank of the creek at it winds northeast. You cross to the north bank at 16.9 miles and continue north through a copse of mesquite trees. Climb steeply around and then on top of the ridge, where the vegetation has been reduced to tall grass, small juniper, and the ubiquitous prickly pear. Toward the top of this first ridge, the trail will turn southeast, crossing two washes as it winds across the ridgeline. To your right, you can see the whole of Paradise Canyon plunging down into the confluence.

Past that second wash, you steeply ascend the almost empty hillside, turning east as you go, until you find yourself on top of the ridge at 4,560 feet. The trail descends northward from here, switchbacking steeply into the next ravine, where you will come upon a barbed-wire fence that surrounds the concrete tanks of Frog Tanks Spring.

Stay on Frog Tanks Trail as it bends south alongside the ravine and then up over a little saddle, turning northeast in the process.

Follow the ridgeline along a trail of barbeque-colored lava rock, across a meadow (yes, a real meadow), and then through a stand of widely spaced juniper. At the top, your path reunites with Reavis Ranch Trail.

Reavis Ranch Trail is an abandoned roadway through here that's littered with lava rock. Turn right (southeast). Within 1 mile, the trail narrows to a singletrack as it passes through a ponderosa pine forest. You are entering Reavis Valley, the site of Reavis Ranch, one of the most popular destinations in the eastern Superstitions. Meadows open up to your left, and here and there are the artifacts of civilization: a rotting planter, rusting coils of barbed wire, and the bare foundation of Reavis Cabin, burned to the ground by foolish campers in the 1990s. You're heading nearly due south by now. Past the cabin, the trail crosses a grassy meadow and a popular campsite. Where the dirt track forks, go left to Reavis Creek, the most reliable water source in the area. Straight across that creek is Fireline Trail 118.

Fireline Trail starts as a straight orange scar running up the scrub-covered hillside. At the top of the hill, you'll march through stands of oak, pinon pine, sycamore, and juniper. Farther on, you cross a wooded ravine and then a pleasant meadow.

At your 23-mile mark, look for the cairns marking the Circlestone spur trail. This unofficial spur trail is better laid out and maintained than earlier material might indicate. It starts as a steep series of switchbacks but then levels out as you cross the top of the ridgeline toward the southern prominence where the site lies, some 0.75 miles from Fireline Trail.

Here you'll discover a low circular wall constructed of loose stones, built by the Salado for unknown reasons—though perhaps the view was a factor in selecting the site. You're not supposed to camp here, but that restriction is obviously widely ignored. When you have satisfied your curiosity, backtrack to the Fireline and continue right up the next ridge. Past the top, at 5,380 feet, follow the plummeting switchbacks (you lose nearly 1,200 feet in just over 1 mile), descending out of transition scrub and into pine forest as you go. Deer of all sizes and even elk have been seen in this canyon; you'll have almost certainly noticed black bear scat on the trail.

Just shy of 27 miles, you cross Campaign Creek to reach the intersection with Campaign Trail, and a flat, pine tree–lined plain where you can make your next camp.

The third leg starts southwest (right from the Fireline junction), down the south bank of Campaign Creek. In less than 1 mile, you come to your first crossing—it's a tricky one. Double back 100 feet or so to find the cairns. The trail across goes sharply back to the right (roughly north) to begin a long, winding climb over the bluff. You have little chance of finding this path by bushwhacking, so make certain you locate the cairns.

Campaign Trail winds up Campaign Creek until it eventually leaves the drainage to climb over the saddle. Arizona sycamore, pine, spruce, and oak all populate these woods, but the species you encounter most is the manzanita, whose red- and gray-striped branches frequently reach across the trail.

Crossing the drainage may require acrobatics, especially higher in the canyon. Other than these treacherous crossings, and the overly affectionate manzanita, the path is a moderate grade along often shaded packed-dirt singletrack.

At 28.5 miles, you leave the creek bed to start climbing out. Yes, go through the bushes as the cairn implies. That really is the trail. Happily, the switchbacks aren't as obstructed all the way, but they are steep.

At the top of the saddle, at 5,300 feet, you pass through a gate (close it behind you). Pinto Peak pokes up above the ridgeline to your left. This slope is all chaparral as you descend south, via steep, rocky switchbacks. The trail follows the ridgeline, and the fence on top of it, winding southeast. Below, you can make out Oak Flats, at the confluence of four canyons. Sawtooth Ridge towers ahead, across those canyons to the south.

Just shy of 30 miles, you must open and close another gate. A mile later, the switchbacks start in earnest, leading you down past the chocolate-covered rock formations you've been looking at all the way down. Past this formation, the switchbacks are closer together and steeper as the juniper forest closes in. When the path levels out, you have returned to Oak Flats. Continue south across the sycamore- and oak-shaded meadow. To your left, as you near Pinto Creek, is a circular wooden fence held together by bailing wire and cowboy engineering. Across the stream is your intersection with West Pinto Trail. Go left (east) on that trail to return to the Miles trailhead.

DIRECTIONS: From Apache Junction, take US 60 east 44 miles passing Superior and a small community called "Top-o-the-World." Turn left on Pinto Valley Road (FR 287) between mileposts 239 and 240. This road is a partially paved maze through giant mining operations. The mining companies' willingness to move whole hills around makes maps useless, but they have put up many signs stating which road is public and which roads definitely are not. Take your time and pay attention, and you should find your way through.

Follow this route about 6.5 miles to FR 287A, an intersection marked by a large sycamore tree and a car-camping area. This dirt road has a reasonable grade but many rocks and ruts. You need a medium- or higher-clearance vehicle past this point. Turn left and wind up into the canyons on this road for 5.5 miles; it will seem longer. The road dead-ends at Miles trailhead, on the site of an old ranch.

Near the parking area, a cattle pen and a small shed still stand. Large sycamore and oak trees shade the lot, making this an excellent area for car camping. However, there are no services.

GPS Trailhead Coordinates	12 EASTERN SUPERSTITIONS SUPERLOOP
UTM zone (WGS 84)	12S
Easting	493718
Northing	3699801
Latitude/Longitude	
North	33° 26' 15.3"
West	111° 04' 03.3"

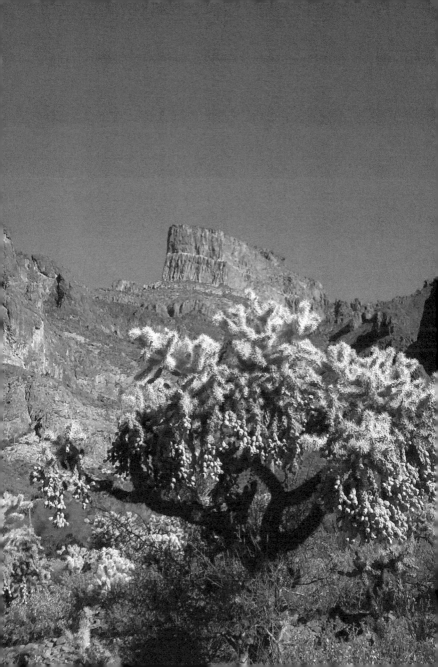

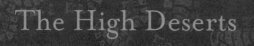

The High Deserts

3

Explore
numerous
high peaks,
deep gorges,
babbling
river
beds,
near-silent
deserts,
hundred-
year-old
mining
camps,
or thousand-
year-old
Native
American
settlements

SCENERY: ☆ ☆ ☆	DISTANCE: *8.6 miles*
TRAIL CONDITION: ☆ ☆ ☆	HIKING TIME: *4 hours*
CHILDREN: ☆ ☆ ☆	OUTSTANDING FEATURES: *Riparian area,*
DIFFICULTY: ☆	*running water, crowned saguaro cacti*
SOLITUDE: ☆ ☆	

This hike follows the perennial Cave Creek through its lush riparian upper course then cuts around some desert hills to rejoin the river lower in its canyon. This trail is both scenic and easy year-round. The estimated hike time assumes you spend some time splashing around. This stretch is the most popular of the Cave Creek trail system.

🚶🚶 Starting at the Cave Creek trailhead, climb Trail 4 up the hill and follow it as it heads south, past the campground. It will dip back down soon, to a fork. To your left is an unmarked trail to the campground. Go right, heading back south up the hill.

In less than 1 mile, the trail descends to cross FR 248 (which leads to the Ashdale administrative site). Go straight across. Soon the trail splits again. To the left is the equestrian bypass; the main route, to your right, goes over a barbed-wire fence via metal stairs. The equestrian bypass goes down the hill, through a gate, and then back up to join the main trail. Since the main route is shorter, stay right.

As you descend into Cave Creek Canyon, the scrub juniper you have been hiking through will yield to larger trees—maple, cottonwood, and elm shade the trail. Soon you will come to a sign announcing a junction with Cottonwood Trail 247. Stay to the right, on Trail 4, and you will see a barbed-wire fence, and beyond that, the scrub juniper ecosystem that separates the desert from the forest. To your left, Cave Creek babbles on and off behind the huge cottonwood and sycamore trees that line its bank. After about 1 mile, you'll come to a cattle gate near Big Maggie May wash, which is normally dry.

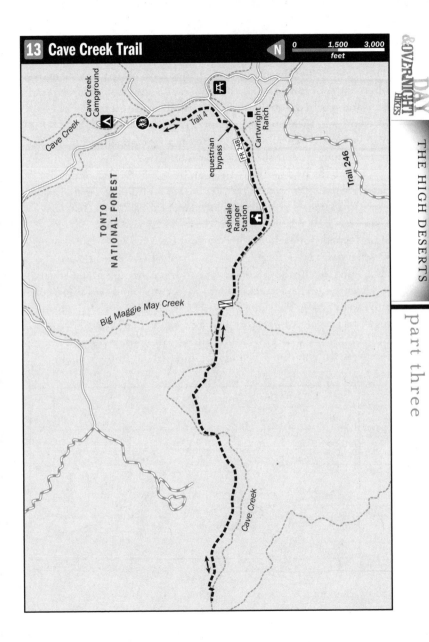

0   1,500   3,000
feet

Cave Creek Campground

Cave Creek

TONTO NATIONAL FOREST

Trail 4

equestrian bypass

FR 248

Cartwright Ranch

Ashdale Ranger Station

Trail 246

Big Maggie May Creek

Cave Creek

Across the wash, the trail narrows as it passes between some huge boulders. That's when you need to find a way across Cave Creek. This is the first of three crossings. A rock cairn on the far side marks where the trail continues. It is possible, of course, to ignore the trail here and stay in the streambed. This would require a fair bit of bush-whacking and rock-hopping and perhaps some wading if the water is high enough. The trail will return to the stream in about 1 mile. If you wish to keep your shoes dry, stay on the trail.

Climb the trail up the ridge. You'll soon be in high Sonoran desert, with all the cacti and sticker bushes found there, including some fine samples of acacia and buckhorn cholla. While Cave Creek takes a leisurely northward bend, the trail cuts across the ridge, almost exactly following the 3,400-foot line on a topographic map. On the west side of the ridge, the trail switchbacks down toward the river, hugging the canyon wall about 75 feet above the stream until it descends into the riverbed. This will be the second crossing. Signs and cairns render the route fairly obvious. If the water level is at all high, deep pools will form along the creek. A good variety of native fish—long-finned dace, Gila and fathead minnows, and green sunfish are among the more prominent—swim about in these pools.

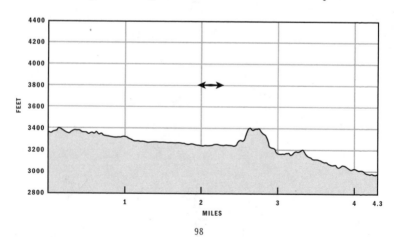

On the other side, the trail heads up another 100 feet, hugging the canyon wall some more. The slopes of Cramm Mountain, to your right, are guarded by old, fat, happy saguaros and pancake prickly pears. Keep an eye out for some rare crowned saguaros. You'll go through them past Cramm Mountain and the peak on the far side of the creek. After 1 mile of this, you descend once more toward the creek.

Cave Creek rolls over some large, blue boulders here, and the grassy banks are dotted with mesquite trees. This is your turnaround point for the day hike. The trail itself crosses the creek, goes another 6 miles, and loses nearly 900 feet in elevation before terminating at Skull Mesa trailhead (see hike 19, page 125). Take some time to take a dip in the cool water. Return the way you came.

DIRECTIONS: Follow Cave Creek Road north from Phoenix, all the way through Cave Creek and then Carefree, until you pass the ranger station. Soon after this, Cave Creek Road becomes Forest Road 24. Follow this winding, partially paved road about 13 miles, until you come to Seven Springs Recreation Area. Within this area you will pass a picnic area and the Civilian Conservation Corps campground. At that point, watch for the trailhead on your left. Cave Creek trailhead has paved parking, a picnic table, vault toilets, and an engraved wooden sign displaying all the trails you can access from this point.

GPS Trailhead Coordinates 13 CAVE CREEK TRAIL
UTM zone (WGS 84) 12S
Easting 0420020
Northing 3759240
Latitude/Longitude
North 33° 58' 21.4"
West 111° 51' 59.8"

14 Skunk Tank Loop

SCENERY: 🌲 🌲	DISTANCE: *11 miles*
TRAIL CONDITION: 🌲 🌲 🌲	HIKING TIME: *6.5 hours*
CHILDREN: 🌲	OUTSTANDING FEATURES: *Riparian area,*
DIFFICULTY: 🌲 🌲 🌲	*desert vistas, historic route*
SOLITUDE: 🌲 🌲 🌲	

This hike climbs across the mountains, through the ghost manzanitas, and along the old cattle route up to Skunk Tank. It then switchbacks steeply down to the perennial Cave Creek, which it follows back uphill to form a loop. The route offers great views of the surrounding mountains and canyons and a perspective on the history of the area and what has been lost.

🚶🚶 Staring at the Cave Creek trailhead, climb Trail 4 up the hill and follow it as it heads south, past the campground. In less than 1 mile, the trail descends to cross FR 248 (which leads to the Ashdale administrative site). Go straight across. Shortly after that, the trail splits again. To the left is the equestrian bypass. The main route, on your right, goes over a barbed-wire fence via metal stairs. The equestrian bypass goes down the hill, through a gate, and then back up to join the main trail. Since the main route is shorter, stay right.

Soon you come to a sign announcing a junction with Cottonwood Trail 247. That trail, which is the one you want, crosses Cave Creek. You'll have to find your way through the maze of saplings midway through the streambed, but once you're through them, more cairns will show the way—or, at least, someone's opinion of the way. Look left, upstream, for the ramp trail leading out of the streambed.

This northern tip of the Cottonwood Trail skirts Cartwright Ranch, which is still an active enterprise. This well-used trail has a gentle grade through here, and traffic has worn it down to a trough through soft dirt. In less than 1 mile, you'll come to the junction

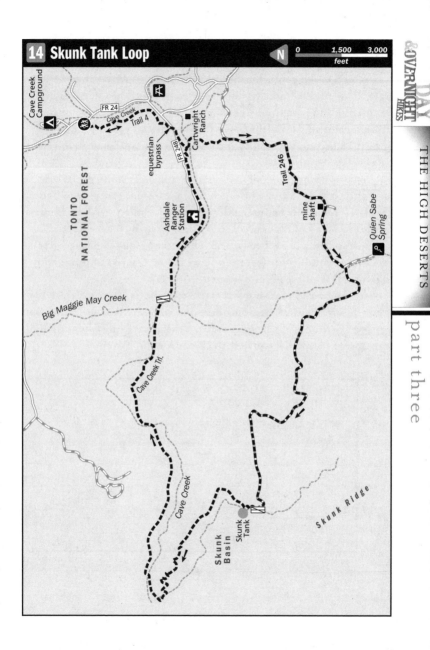

14 Skunk Tank Loop

N

0   1,500   3,000
feet

DAY
& OVERNIGHT
HIKES

Cave Creek Campground

FR 24

Cave Creek
Trail 4

Cartwright Ranch

equestrian bypass

FR 248

Trail 246

Ashdale Ranger Station

mine shaft

Quien Sabe Spring

TONTO
NATIONAL FOREST

Big Maggie May Creek

Cave Creek Trl.

Cave Creek

Skunk Tank

Skunk Basin

Skunk Ridge

with Trail 246, which leads to Skunk Tank. Turn right, more south than east, up this trail.

You'll climb gently but steadily through juniper scrub terrain then enter the area recently ravaged by fire. The skeletons of manzanita and ironwood trees haunt the trail—ghosts of the once-thick scrubland. But at the base of most of them, you'll see new growth. Keep your eyes out for a craterous old mineshaft to the right (downslope) of the trail.

By this point, the trail has widened in places, revealing its origins as a cattle trail: the route by which ranchers lead their cattle to Skunk Tank. Infrequently maintained, parts of this cattle track have become badly eroded, and rocks of all sizes litter the path. Whereas the hills around you are mostly brown and yellow, with isolated dabs of green, the rocks beneath your feet show more color. Chunks of pearly white quartz and sky-blue granite decorate the trail.

You'll have to pick your way across some holes where the track has washed away; many of the slopes have eroded down to bare granite. But the level portions, which typify much of this route, are of soft dirt and easy going, except that you have to climb from time to time.

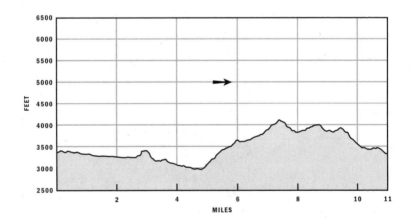

At the top of this climb, you'll come to the junction with Quien Sabe Trail 250. A number of recent signs replace the one whose burnt post remains. Stay on Skunk Trail, which descends from here, toward the tank itself. As you close in on the tank, rock cairns, some more necessary than others, mark the trail. The tank holds plenty of water after a rain but more often is a wide, flat crater of mud. The banks are choked with thistles. Go through the cattle gate (closing it behind you) and down into the wash below the tank. A thicket of brush blocks the wash, forming the downstream edge of Skunk Tank. Here you'll find abundant shade, green grass, and even some rocks to sit on.

On the far side of the wash, the trail crosses a saddle while bending north. Here and there you will notice the skeletons of once-mighty saguaro cacti—victims of recent fires. Fire is not normal in the Sonoran desert, and most species have not adapted to it. It can take more than 50 years for native species to recover following a fire. Unfortunately, exotic species, particularly grasses introduced from Africa or southern Europe, respond well to fire and tend to displace the native species after a burn.

Less than 1 mile past the wash, the trail will start its infamous descent into Cave Creek Canyon, switchbacking from 4,000 feet at the tank to 2,900 feet at Cave Creek in less than 2 miles. Soon, you will know what your knees are made of. The trail is very narrow in places and crosses exposed and slippery granite. Take your time. At the bottom, the trail reaches a T-intersection with Cave Creek Trail. Go right (east) to head upstream. This is your route back to the trailhead.

Cave Creek Trail is a lovely stroll that alternates between lush riparian thickets and stark Sonoran hillsides (see hike 13 on page 96). What you need to know is that you'll cross the stream three times; all crossings are reasonably well marked with cairns. You'll follow this trail about 3 miles, until you reencounter the signed junction with Cottonwood Trail. From here, continue back along Trail 4 to the trailhead.

DIRECTIONS: Follow Cave Creek Road north from Phoenix, all the way through Cave Creek and then Carefree, until you pass the ranger station. Soon after this, Cave Creek Road becomes Forest Road 24. Follow this winding, partially paved road about 13 miles until you come to the Seven Springs Recreation Area. Within this area you will pass a picnic area and the Civilian Conservation Corps campground. At that point, watch for the trailhead on your left: there's paved parking, a picnic table, vault toilets, and an engraved wooden sign displaying all the trails you can access from this point.

GPS Trailhead Coordinates	14 SKUNK TANK LOOP
UTM zone (WGS 84)	12S
Easting	0420020
Northing	3759240
Latitude/Longitude	
North	33° 58' 21.4"
West	111° 51' 59.8"

SCENERY: ☆ ☆ ☆ ☆	DISTANCE: *11 miles*
TRAIL CONDITION: ☆ ☆ ☆	HIKING TIME: *5.5 hours*
CHILDREN: ☆ ☆ ☆	OUTSTANDING FEATURES: *Transition desert,*
DIFFICULTY: ☆ ☆ ☆	*an old cabin, and boulders upon boulders; in spring,*
SOLITUDE: ☆ ☆ ☆	*running creeks and abundant wildflowers*

This hike follows Pine Creek Trail to Ballantine Trail then climbs to a cutoff for an unofficial trail to an old cabin. An even more unofficial trail leads you back over the ridge to rejoin the Ballantine, which you follow back to the trailhead. The route over the hill to the cabin and back is steep and sometimes hard to follow, but it's worth it. Along the way, you will see plenty of cool rock formations, but in spring, all the pretty flowers will vie for your attention.

🚶🚶 From the Ballantine trailhead, Pine Creek Loop 280 presents you with a choice. To your right, the trail goes east, switchbacking straight up and over the cactus-covered hill. To your left, it winds gently around the hill. Go left.

You ascend north at an easy grade through upper Sonoran vegetation, highlighted by majestic, multiarmed saguaros. After 1 mile, the trail has wound eastward, the roar of AZ 87 dies away, and you can hear Pine Creek babbling some 300 feet below. The trail hugs the southern slope of this hill and keeps climbing, pulling away from Pine Creek until it turns southward, up the saddle. Here you'll find the junction with Ballantine Trail. A sign at the junction indicates distances to various landmarks but does not mention the 1,000-foot elevation gain necessary to reach them. Go straight (east) toward the boulder-covered hills.

Soon you start switchbacking through the boulders on a steep track that is occasionally eroded down to bare, slick sandstone. At

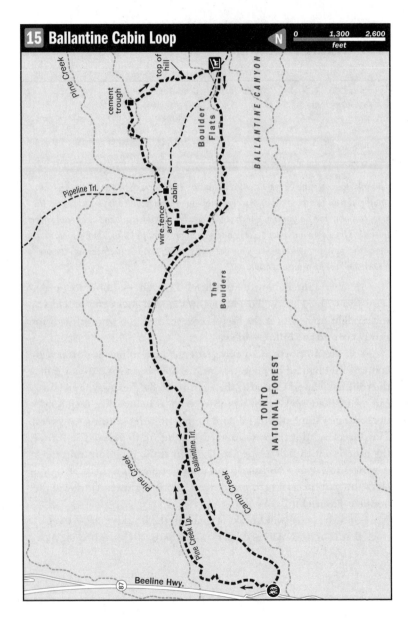

15 Ballantine Cabin Loop

N

0   1,300   2,600
feet

Pine Creek

top of hill

BALLANTINE CANYON

cement trough

Boulder Flats

Pipeline Trl.

wire fence   cabin
arch

The Boulders

TONTO
NATIONAL FOREST

Pine Creek

Ballantine Trl.

Cavan Creek

Pine Creek Lp.

Beeline Hwy.

87

the top of this trudge, about 1 mile farther and 600 feet higher, the trail will level out for a spell, winding past some enormous boulders. Camp Creek flows down the canyon to your right.

After a couple of additional short climbs and past the barbed-wire fence, the trail winds close to Camp Creek and then winds away again as it ascends. At about 3.6 miles in, you'll come to a trail junction. To your right is an enormous formation of boulders crowning a low hill. To your left is a narrow trail wandering off toward a ridge to the north. At your feet you'll see the trail sign: its singed remains are held in place with a couple of rocks. It won't mention the cabin trail to the north. Take that left anyway. The side trail makes a steep, gravelly ascent and then a steeper descent on the far side of the hill. Go through the barbed-wire archway, then continue east down the fence and head through the catclaws to the cabin.

The corrugated-tin structure has a picnic bench, a ruined stove, and a random assortment of discarded camping supplies and canned food. The hole in the dirt floor and the scat on the table testify that this may be a lively spot for vermin at night. A barbed-wire fence encircles the yard, except where you came in and where a jeep trail goes

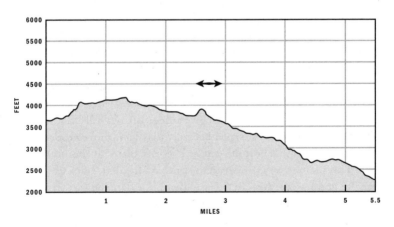

out and to the north. This is a popular trek for 4WD enthusiasts.

Follow the fence line to the right of the jeep trail to find a narrow trail continuing east. This trail has been made, or at least reinforced, by dirt bikes. It winds in and out of the wash through the high desert prairie surrounded by huge, gray boulders and a scattering of quartz. Follow the narrow track about 1.5 miles, until it comes to a concrete cattle tank.

The trail goes south from here, up the drainage and then straight over the boulder-covered hill. Once you are out of the drainage and going up the hill itself, the trail becomes very steep, and your predecessors have had differing opinions as to how to get around various obstacles. So long as you keep climbing, though, you'll find that all the spurs come together at the top of the hill, at just over 4,000 feet elevation.

Rock cairns guide you on the gentle descent down the other side, where, after about 0.25 miles, you will come to an old corral and the junction with the Ballantine Trail. You have journeyed just under 6 miles at this point.

If you go left through the corral, you'll see that the Ballantine continues east, where it will eventually reach 5,800 feet on its climb around Pine Mountain, and then descend precariously to the distant Cline trailhead. Taking that route would add two orders of difficulty to this hike. Turning right (west), the Ballantine crosses Boulder Flats before descending down toward where you came from.

The even, dirt trail wanders among a scattering of mesquite trees, some still showing fire damage. The barbed-wire fence marks the start of a rough passage through boulder-strewn hills. Soon the trail will descend more sharply, becoming rockier, more eroded, and more treacherous. It bottoms out in a second plain, at about 3,600 feet. This plain is very similar to the one you just left, but with more needles and fewer leaves. In the middle of this flat, you will cross Camp Creek. At the west end of it, you will return to the junction where you went north to seek the cabin.

Now, of course, you go straight (west), the way you came back to the trailhead.

DIRECTIONS: From Fountain Hills (in the northeast corner of the Phoenix metro area), go about 26 miles north on AZ 87. You'll see the sign for the trailhead just past mile marker 210. The trailhead is a graded dirt circle drive with no services, though a large sign marks the start of the trail.

GPS Trailhead Coordinates	15 BALLANTINE CABIN LOOP
UTM zone (WGS 84)	12S
Easting	454298.07
Northing	3736132.54
Latitude/Longitude	
North	33° 45' 51.5"
West	111° 29' 36.7"

SCENERY: ✿ ✿ ✿ ✿	DISTANCE: *8.5 miles*
TRAIL CONDITION: ✿ ✿	HIKING TIME: *4 hours 45 minutes*
CHILDREN: ✿ ✿	OUTSTANDING FEATURES: *Three different*
DIFFICULTY: ✿ ✿ ✿	*vegetation zones, box canyon, horse corral, riparian*
SOLITUDE: ✿ ✿ ✿	*glades, part of the Arizona Trail (AZT)*

This hike near Lake Roosevelt marches up Cottonwood Canyon, wandering back and forth between three different vegetation zones (upper Sonoran, transition scrub, and riparian). After climbing the canyon, the trail follows a forest road up the slopes and then reenters the upper canyon to access a truly remarkable stand of riparian hardwoods. This route is part of the Arizona Trail, which runs from Mexico to Utah. Do not confuse this with Cottonwood Trail 256 near Cave Creek.

🚶🚶 The Frazier trailhead is immediately behind the Frazier substation. Just past the trailhead is a 0.5-mile spur trail leading to Frazier Campground (sense a theme here?). Stay on the main trail, which goes south a bit but then winds west, going over and around a couple of ridges before turning south again and descending into Cottonwood Creek Canyon proper. You'll see excellent specimens of prickly pear and palo verde trees along this stretch. On the far side of the canyon is a trailer park and access to Cemetery Trail, which does, in fact, lead to an old cemetery.

Staying on the Cottonwood, you'll travel along a fence, past a small water tank, and then through a gate. Close the gate behind you. You're going south and uphill into the canyon. Within 1 mile of the gate, the steep red and pink walls of the canyon start to close in. In the morning light, this provides an excellent photo opportunity: a small slice of Sedona, without the trouble, expense, or spiritual agitation.

The trail crosses the creek bed several times through here. Tall rock piles will mark the way through red and pink boulders. The

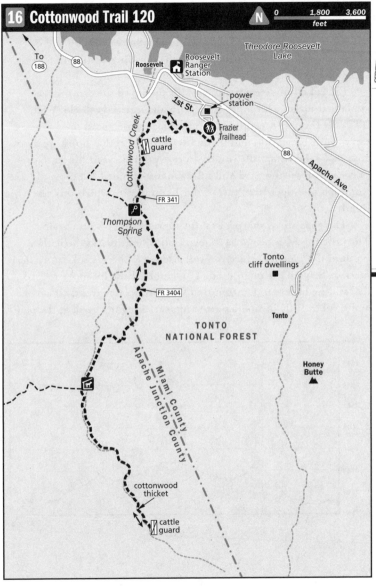

16 Cottonwood Trail 120

N   0   1,800   3,600
         feet

DAY &OVERNIGHT HIKES

THE HIGH DESERTS

part three

To (188)

(88)

Roosevelt

Roosevelt Ranger Station

Theodore Roosevelt Lake

power station

1st St.

Frazier Trailhead

(88)

Apache Ave.

Cottonwood Creek

cattle guard

FR 341

Thompson Spring

FR 3404

Tonto cliff dwellings

Tonto

TONTO NATIONAL FOREST

Honey Butte

Miami County

Apache Junction County

cottonwood thicket

cattle guard

canyon will widen, though, as you see the cottonwood trees ahead of you. Beneath these trees, Forest Road 341 crosses Cottonwood Creek and intersects your trail. The forest road is your route up and out of the canyon. Follow it straight (south), heading uphill—not west across the streambed.

FR 341 climbs steeply and steadily up out of the canyon at a grade that makes a lot more sense with a motorized vehicle. Well, it's really three consecutive hard climbs. A cattle guard marks the top of your last climb, and if you turn around at that point, you can appreciate the vista while you try to re-oxygenate your blood. Not only can you see the road and hills you just climbed but most of Lake Roosevelt and the better part of the Tonto Basin, which this reservoir floods.

The road turns sharply west for a stretch, then south again. The junction with FR 3404, a jeep trail at best, marks the halfway point of the journey. Here you will also see a fiberglass Arizona Trail marker. Stay on the main road. You climb a little bit more before descending back into Cottonwood Canyon. Joshua trees, saguaros, and scrubby little junipers start to appear along this road as the palo

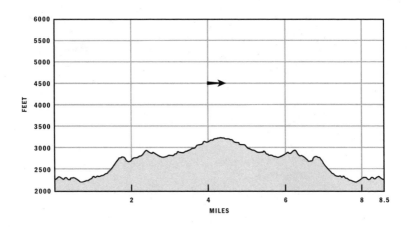

verde starts to disappear. As it dips, the road passes a large water tank and a corral. This is where you exit, for on the far side of the corral is the continuation of Trail 120. You'll find another AZT blaze and a sign warning that, due to recent flooding, the trail beyond is not recommended for horses.

Follow the trail roughly south from here as it runs along a barbed-wire fence and the thin water pipe that feeds the cattle tank. Several discarded lengths of pipe also litter the trail. Soon after you wander through stands of mesquite surrounded by stands of saguaro, you'll cross the wash, leaving fence and pipe behind. The farther you go upstream, the better your chance of encountering running water. Within 1 mile, you'll cross again and may be rock-hopping to keep your boots dry. Here you rejoin the pipeline but not the fence.

Soon, though, the trail will leave the pipe to hug a cliff wall and then cross the stream yet again. Trees, real trees—oak, maple, birch, and the eponymous cottonwood—tower over the riverbed now. But this also begins the portion of the trail the sign warned you about. The path picks its way through rocks and driftwood, around huge trees, through thickets of saplings, and occasionally up steep embankments that may require you use all four limbs to scramble up (and perhaps your keester to scramble down). It goes on like this for a good mile, and any spot you pick to rest and regroup is going to be a pretty one. That spot will also be a good turnaround spot, unless you can't get enough of the high desert landscape that awaits on the other side of these riparian woods.

Beyond the big trees, the trail climbs farther up the canyon and into open desert once again. There is a cattle gate about 0.5 miles beyond (from which this hike distance is calculated). The trail continues though this terrain for 1 mile or so until it hits Forest Road 83.

DIRECTIONS: From Phoenix, take AZ 87, Beeline Highway, north to AZ 188. From Mesa take AZ 88, Apache Trail, north to AZ 188. In either case, take AZ 188 past the dam (and across the bridge near the dam to Forest Road 173). The turnoff is immediately before the power substation, a couple miles past the bridge. You pass the trailer park on your right, the ranger station to your left, cross Cottonwood Creek, and then look for the turn on your right (all of these landmarks are fairly close together). If you reach Tonto National Monument, you've gone too far. Frazier trailhead is a graded dirt circle drive with no services and requires no fee.

GPS Trailhead Coordinates	16 COTTONWOOD TRAIL 120
UTM zone (WGS 84)	12S
Easting	0488580
Northing	3724550
Latitude/Longitude	
North	33° 39' 41.6"
West	111° 7' 24.0"

17 Picketpost Mountain Trail

SCENERY: ⭐ ⭐ ⭐ ⭐	DISTANCE: *4.45 miles*
TRAIL CONDITION: ⭐ ⭐	HIKING TIME: *4.5 hours*
CHILDREN: ⭐	OUTSTANDING FEATURES: *Big and weird*
DIFFICULTY: ⭐ ⭐ ⭐ ⭐	*cacti, extraordinary views, cool rock formations, and*
SOLITUDE: ⭐ ⭐	*a little red mailbox full of thoughts*

This challenging climb scrambles up and through two Sonoran ecosystems to the top of Picketpost Mountain. There you'll find a panoramic view of the entire southern Tonto, plus a little red mailbox. The trail up this mountain is not an official Forest Service trail and requires some route finding and a fair bit of guts.

🚶🚶 From the Picketpost trailhead, you'll start south on the Arizona Trail (AZT), whose passage through the trailhead parking lot is well marked. This recently improved section crosses a couple of washes before intersecting a jeep trail. At the jeep trail, less than 1 mile into the hike, leave the AZT and go left (east). The jeep road winds straight up the hills toward the mountain until it dead-ends at the secondary trailhead for the summit trail about 1 mile past the parking lot.

A concrete slab lies before a wooden post, which once hosted a sign indicating the trail up the mountain. A narrow trail goes straight from that post and across the ravine, but the more obvious trail, going straight up the slope from the post, is the one you want. This switchback route is a little easier on the knees and traverses some very fine cacti. The routes will join before the serious climbing begins.

It is worth stressing here that neither of these trails is an official Forest Service trail. They were blazed and maintained by your fellow hikers and do not always follow the logic that Forest Service trail engineers (or their insurance lawyers) prefer. You'll be hard pressed to tell the difference at first, for the well-defined track picks its way

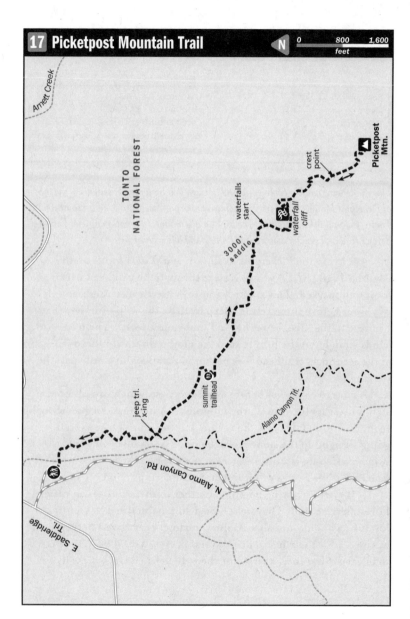

N

0   800   1,600
feet

Arnett Creek

TONTO
NATIONAL FOREST

crest
point

Picketpost
Mtn.

waterfalls
start

waterfall
cliff

3000'
saddle

jeep trl.
x-ing

summit
trailhead

Alamo Canyon Trl.

N. Alamo Canyon Rd.

E. Saddleridge Trl.

carefully up a ridgeline abounding with cholla, then, a little higher, barrel cacti as tall as yourself, and saguaros as tall as anything that grows in the desert.

Toward the top of the ridge, the trail comes to a saddle (where the alternate trail will join it). This spot, at about 3,000 feet elevation, and 1.3 miles from the trailhead, is where you stow your walking stick. The trail past here becomes steep enough that you will need your hands (and occasionally your knees) to clamber up. If you or any member of your party is not comfortable with that, turn around.

From here on out, if in doubt, assume the route heads straight up. Yes, really, straight up. For example, the slab of bare granite right in front of you? You climb straight up that. Every once in while, and more frequently as you near the top, you'll see spray-painted arrows or dots. The white arrows seem to have been made by someone on their way up, whereas the red ones were clearly made by someone on the way down. Regardless of what you think about the environmental impact of such markings, they do make the way easier to find, especially in spots where scrambling about could prove disastrous. Climb the steep, rocky switchbacks up the lower slopes

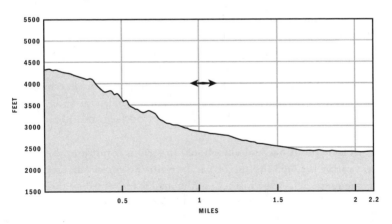

of the mountain. The term "goat-trail" would only glorify the route through here. There are a couple of places where you will hug the cliff-side like a dear, dear friend.

Soon you will come to a point where water flows across the trail. This could be a stream, falls, ice, a seep, or a stain depending on the temperature and recent rainfall. Any level of wetness makes the rhyolite slopes extremely slippery, so the more you can keep the bottoms of your boots dry, the better off you are.

Pick your way past the seeps until you come to the sheer cliff side, with water flowing down through a couple slots and paint-marks that seem to contradict each other. That slick, steep surface is, in fact, your best route up. How exactly you climb it depends upon your nerves, your height, and how much confidence you have in the traction of your soles. There's about 50 feet of scariness, and then the arrows begin to agree upon a single route. Take heart—according to the log at the top, this route has been traversed by senior citizens, dogs, and by one account, a five-year-old girl.

The trail now switchbacks through a thicket of cane cholla, with various branches waving wildly westward, as if blown by a wind felt only by the cacti. This thin trail is plenty steep, but well defined, and can be traversed using mostly just your feet. It continues to wind up through decaying pillars of basalt as you near the crest of the mountain.

The crest of the mountain is flat, like the top of a mesa. A trail leads you across the yucca and century plants, knee-high grass, and crumbling basalt to the actual peak itself, a mound of rocks crowned with a bright-red mailbox. When you reach this point, at 4,347 feet elevation, you will have climbed just over 1,900 feet in a little more than 2 miles.

The mailbox has several logbooks in various conditions. Sign in. Leafing through the entries can be quite the exercise in amateur archaeology. The "true history" of the mailbox is inscribed inside the lid. A Superior resident, one of your fellow hikers who helped blaze the summit route, hauled it up here in 1994.

As you return the way you came, remember that keeping your keester in contact with the cliff will help slow your descent.

DIRECTIONS: Take US 60 east from Mesa. Turn off on FR 231 just past Mile Marker 221. Watch out for construction. If you reach Queen Creek Bridge, you've gone too far. Proceed down the graded dirt road to the signed left turn onto a paved road. This will dead-end in 0.6 miles at the Picketpost trailhead, which has vaulted toilets but no other facilities. A caretaker works in season, fall to spring. US 60 is being expanded through here, so these directions may change.

GPS Trailhead Coordinates	17 PICKETPOST MOUNTAIN TRAIL
UTM zone (WGS 84)	12S
Easting	483542.25
Northing	3681501.66
Latitude/Longitude	
North	N 33° 16' 20.7"
West	W 111° 10' 36.2"

SCENERY: ⛰ ⛰	DISTANCE: *6 miles*
TRAIL CONDITION: ⛰ ⛰	HIKING TIME: *3 hours*
CHILDREN: ⛰ ⛰	OUTSTANDING FEATURES: *Scenic vistas of the*
DIFFICULTY: ⛰	*New River Mountains, transition eco-zone, quartz*
SOLITUDE: ⛰ ⛰ ⛰ ⛰	*and mica, isolation*

This hike follows the rough remains of Forest Road 602 to the start of Trail 8, one of the most isolated and least documented trails on the Tonto map. The hike then follows that trail to the first saddle, beyond which recent fires have made travel more trouble than it's worth.

🚶 FR 602 intersects with FR 24 across a sandstone saddle marked by a nearby chimney-rock formation called CP Butte. Unless you have a serious 4WD, this is the start of your hike. Even if you do have a suitable vehicle, your likely top speed is 5 mph on much of the upcoming road. Save the tires and hike.

FR 602 crosses a wash, goes through a gate (all within sight of your vehicle), and then becomes a wide bed of stumble-rocks climbing steeply up the ridge for the next mile. Not an easy stretch to take by Jeep or foot. At the top of the ridge, as the road becomes a gentler dirt track, you pass a campsite to your right. Cross the ridge and make the gentle, if rocky, descent down the other side. You'll pass an unmarked side road. Stay on 602 as it winds in and out of a ravine, turning more northward as it does so.

Classic transition scrub begins around 4,000 feet, with yucca and prickly pear representing the last of the high desert, and juniper and manzanita representing the first of the lower forest. Tall prairie grass grows all around, along with a lot of catclaw—but it's not such a problem when you're walking on the road.

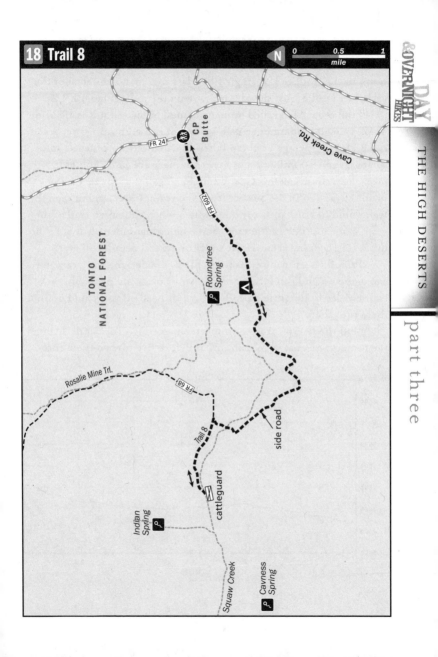

N

0   0.5   1
mile

CP Butte

FR 24

Cave Creek Rd.

FR 602

TONTO
NATIONAL FOREST

Roundtree
Spring

Rosalie Mine Trl.

FR 68

Trail 8

side road

cattleguard

Indian
Spring

Cavness
Spring

Squaw Creek

Follow the road north along the eastern slopes of two bramble-covered hills before crossing a drainage and then climbing a little more to the trailhead. A single fiberglass sign marks the start of the reclusive Trail 8, just shy of 3 miles from the pulloff from FR 24.

Trail 8 has been called by many names. Some call it Rosalie Mine Trail, though it does not actually go to that ruined mining site. Some call it Hogan Springs Trail (and there is a theoretical route to those springs, some 10 miles west of here, but there are easier routes to take). You could call this Goat Camp Springs Trail, for that is the major attraction in the Squaw Creek Canyon it traverses, but then the trail would be constantly confused with a more publicized trail of the same name just west of Phoenix. Some older maps identify it as FR 68, but it clearly hasn't seen vehicle traffic in several decades—if ever.

Trail 8, as uninspired as it might be, is a designation everyone can agree on and can locate on any map. You could probably park two vehicles in the little pulloff by the trailhead—if you could bounce them into there.

Find the narrow trail to your left; it ascends a rocky hill through the remains of what were manzanitas before fire turned them into

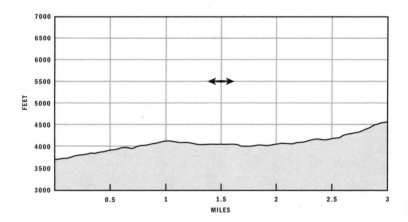

the white skeletons that now dot the hillside. Once you round the corner, heading more west, the hillside greens with undamaged manzanita, juniper, yucca, prickly pear, and sawgrass. This pattern repeats itself a couple of times as you round the hill. Quartz and even flakes of mica glitter amid the chunks of lava rock on the trail. In spring the hillside is adorned with purple and orange flowers.

The trail crosses in and out of a couple of drainages as it winds steeply up the hillside to emerge, about 0.5 miles later, on top of a yucca- and century plant–covered saddle. A barbed-wire fence bisects this rise, but fallen brush has created an opening for the trail. The altitude at the fence is 4,525 feet, about 450 feet higher than the trailhead.

Catch your breath, for this is the turnaround point for people who prefer their hikes to be pleasant. Before the recent fires, the remainder of Trail 8 cruised through a lovely, isolated spring-fed riparian area. The springs and the isolation remain, but fire has scorched the trees. The plant that has recovered the quickest is our friend the catclaw, which has overgrown substantial portions of the route, sometimes in jungle-level profusion.

If you want to see riparian zones, take one of the easier, prettier hikes you passed to get here. Meanwhile, there is just you and the wind on this saddle, and probably no one else for a dozen miles in any direction. Return the way you came.

DIRECTIONS: From Phoenix, follow Cave Creek Road north until it becomes FR 24 near the ranger station. Continue another 12 miles. Once past Seven Springs Recreation Area, the road is entirely graded dirt and may be rough across some of the washes; nevertheless, it's passable—with care—for most vehicles. Turn left on the signed FR 602, and park right there on the sandstone saddle, unless your vehicle is robustly 4WD. You'll find no services at this free site.

GPS Trailhead Coordinates	18 TRAIL 8
UTM zone (WGS 84)	12S
Easting	421745.17
Northing	3774329.54
Latitude/Longitude	
North	34° 06' 24.7"
West	111° 50' 54.4"

SCENERY: ✿ ✿ ✿	DISTANCE: *25.8 miles*
TRAIL CONDITION: ✿ ✿ ✿	HIKING TIME: *17 hours (2 days)*
CHILDREN: ✿ ✿ ✿	OUTSTANDING FEATURES: *Riparian glades,*
DIFFICULTY: ✿ ✿ ✿	*mountain vistas, perennial creeks, three different*
SOLITUDE: ✿ ✿ ✿ ✿ ✿	*eco-zones*

This two-day backpacking loop circumnavigates the entire Cave Creek trail system. From Spur Cross trailhead near Carefree, the route follows the rugged Cottonwood Creek Trail (an old cattle route that travels east around the south side of Skull Mesa) then heads up Cottonwood Creek and across a divide before heading north to follow Bronco Creek to its confluence with Cave Creek. The second leg follows the perennial Cave Creek west down its canyon, then cuts across a high butte, dropping to rejoin with Cottonwood Trail. See the note on alternate approaches at the end of the following description.

👣👣 Your hike starts at Spur Cross Conservation Center, a Maricopa County park. Spur Cross features healthy upper Sonoran desert: barrels; big, weird, mutant saguaros; brittlebush—all the usuals. Follow Spur Cross Trail, labeled SX on the free map (it's a remnant dirt road but is still passable by vehicle). Cave Creek proper runs along the trail's right side as you head north toward Tonto Forest. The park is crowded, especially on the weekends, being popular with seniors, dog lovers, and equestrians.

You'll cross Cave Creek 1.25 miles down the road, then cross a cattle guard, the boundary with Tonto National Forest. Past the boundary, Spur Cross Trail becomes FR 48—a jeep trail following the riparian channel of Cave Creek into the hills. You'll cross the creek three times. The second crossing leads to a horse corral, beyond which is County Trail 252, which winds back west then south into the county park. Your third crossing leads to the Skull Mesa

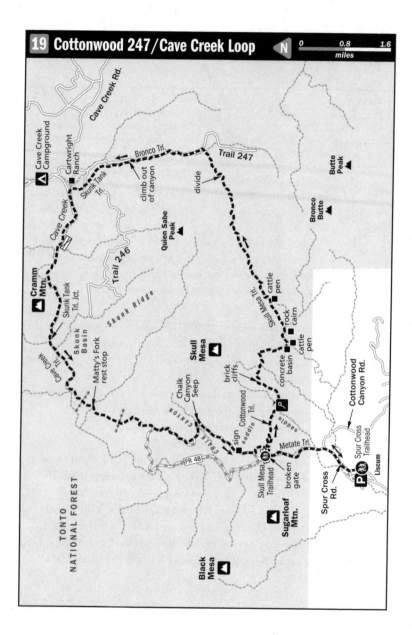

Cave Creek Rd.

Cave Creek Campground

Cartwright Ranch

Bronco Trl.

Trail 247

Butte Peak

Skunk Tank Trl.

climb out of canyon

divide

Bronco Butte

Cave Creek

Cramm Mtn.

Quien Sabe Peak

Trail 246

Skunk Tank Trl. Jct.

Skunk Ridge

Skull Mesa Trl.

cattle pen

rock cairn

cattle pen

Cave Creek Trl.

Skunk Basin

Matty's Fork rest stop

Skull Mesa

concrete basin

brick cliffs

Chalk Canyon Seep

CHALK CANYON

sign

Cottonwood Saddle Trl.

slopes

Cottonwood Canyon Rd.

Metate Trl.

Spur Cross Trailhead

FR 48

Skull Mesa Trailhead

broken gate

Spur Cross Rd.

Liscum

TONTO

NATIONAL FOREST

Sugarloaf Mtn.

Black Mesa

trailhead (mislabeled on some maps as the Spur Cross trailhead), at 2.3 miles in. Take the little road to the right of the sign, FR 1152, to get to the trails. The road to your left will dead-end at a private ranch in about 1 mile.

In a couple hundred yards, the road stops at the intersection of Cave Creek Trail and Cottonwood Trail. Take Cottonwood 246, to the right, immediately crossing the wash. Cottonwood Trail is winding, rugged, and quite beautiful after a rain. This portion doesn't see the sort of traffic that other parts of the trail system endure. Where a clear path has not been pounded, follow the pink nylon ribbons.

You wind up and through orange granite foothills (with attractive lava rock accents) and through upper Sonoran vegetation highlighted by huge stands of prickly pear. You'll notice yucca and juniper crowning the hilltops. A good 500-foot climb takes you to the top of the little saddle, then you descend into a ravine where you cross Cottonwood Springs. Exiting this ravine starts the real climb.

Keep climbing nearly 1,000 feet toward Skull Mesa along a ridgeline. The trail will turn right (east) along a deep ravine opposite startling brick-colored cliffs. Above that canyon, you'll reach the first

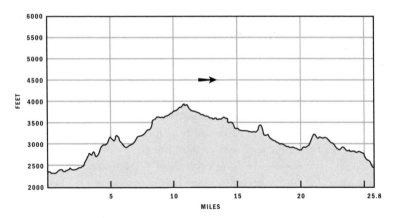

junction with Skull Mesa Trail 248; a sign and a fence announce the intersection. Skull Mesa Trail charges north, straight up the slopes of Skull Mesa. You'll turn south, winding down through an old lava field.

You now follow a historic and still-used cattle trail toward Cottonwood Creek. Soon you'll pass a concrete cattle basin. Go straight, following the barbed-wire fence up the hill and past the little cattle pen. Follow the wide streambed uphill. Like most desert washes, Cottonwood Creek is prone to flash flooding, and this washes out the trail sporadically. The pink ribbons will be a great help, but if the trail seems uncertain, assume it cuts back and forth across the wash. Less than 1 mile later, a rock cairn is visible across a big blue rock formation. The trail remains on the left (north) side of the channel as you head upstream at the fork. You've reached the 3,500-foot line. Juniper becomes more common here, and cactus appears less often.

After 7.7 miles, the trail climbs out of Cottonwood Creek to rendezvous with the other side of Skull Mesa Trail. If you have no interest in that, you can stay in the wash; the trail soon drops back into the canyon. But the juniper-dominated transition scrub makes for a nice change from the mesquite thickets that dominate the wash.

Cottonwood Creek is spring-fed in its upper reaches, and water is relatively reliable, so your many crossings of it may be wet ones. About 1.5 miles after reentering, you climb out of the canyon for good, crossing a 3,900-foot divide to descend into Bronco Creek. Shortly, you come to the intersection with Bronco Trail, a spur to Bronco trailhead, some 3.6 miles farther east. Your trail turns north to follow Bronco Creek down its canyon. In general, the higher, west slope sports juniper-dominated transition scrub, whereas the lower, east slope supports a layer of mesquite with chaparral beyond. Again, where rock cairns fail you, seek pink ribbons.

You stay near Bronco Creek as it flows north toward its confluence with Cave Creek. Before you get there, though, the trail cuts west, across the saddle, becoming as much a trench as a trail in the process. The junction with Skunk Tank Trail means you're getting close. The trail skirts the western boundary of a working ranch before finally crossing Cave Creek to the junction with Cave Creek Trail on the far side. That's right around 14 miles from Spur Cross. Time to make camp.

Less than 1 mile from this junction lies the Civilian Conservation Corps (CCC) campground, which has a $5 fee per vehicle but is free to hikers. It features tables, toilets, and potable water from a pump. If you prefer more primitive and private, your best bet is on the south bank of Cave Creek, opposite the trail.

In the morning, head west down Cave Creek Trail 4. Go through the gate at Maggie May Wash, and cross the perennial stream three times. Just past that third crossing, now on the south bank, you'll come to your second junction with Skunk Tank Trail.

Past this junction, you wind in and out of a wash and then up into a thicket of mesquite, acacia, and a few junipers. The prickly pear starts to predominate here and is a constant presence all the way down. Past this thicket, the trail mows across a grassy bank and then disappears. You're meant to cross the creek here, or at least this fork of it, but the how and where of crossing has been washed away. If you find the way through the brush- and boulder-choked island, follow that. Otherwise follow the stream, and in 0.5 miles or less, the trail will be better marked near where the forks rejoin. This is the only spot on the Cave Creek leg where the trail is not obvious.

About 1 mile later, you pass through an archway in a barbed-wire fence. Past this gate you're in high desert dominated by acacia shrubs and very little shade. Far ahead to the west, you'll see the imposing slopes of New River Mesa. Soon you'll descend into a wash called Matty's Fork, a riparian oasis with oak, maple, and sycamore trees towering over the little babbling brook. You won't pass a better resting place.

Past Matty's Fork, start the serious climb up the bluff, turning south as you go. The higher you climb out of Matty's Fork, the more juniper you see. The trail up the hillside often takes the form of a trench filled with softball-sized lava rocks. High chaparral covers the ridgetop as the trail traces the 3,000-foot line. This singletrack runs through alternating sections of high grass and low grass, according to the whims of desert topology. The soil beneath your boots often has cracks wide enough to swallow a hiking stick. The prickly pear and acacia are now frequently accompanied by cane cholla. Along the trail, you might notice the six-foot-diameter plantations the large red ants have developed. And along the cracked earth, trapdoor spiders have set traps for unwary ants and other prey. This ridge is also popular with lizards, from tiny rock lizards to foot-long Gila monsters (which always have the right of way). On a clear day, keep an eye south so you can see the haze that hovers over Phoenix.

Next you cross a fence line followed by three ravines, each one larger than the last. One is marked by white, then red, then brown soil as you enter it. From the second ravine you can see huge, multi-armed saguaros below you in the distance. The third ravine is, in fact, Chalk Canyon. You cross Chalk Seep, where mesquite trees surround a little seep, and water oozing from the mud trickles down the canyon.

Continue to follow the ridgeline out of Chalk Canyon and across a saddle. As you wind down the saddle, you're in desert proper: orange rock bursts with all the cacti and spiny things characteristic of the lower Sonoran desert. Palo verde replaces the acacia tree, saguaro replaces the juniper, and even the prickly pear yields its place to various forms of cholla.

A fence marks the transition from rocky trail to rocky dirt road. Close the fence if you can—it is in serious need of repair. A short way down this road, you return to the original junction with Cottonwood Trail. You have gone about 9 miles from the junction near the campground. The forest "road" then drops briefly down the hill to the Skull Mesa trailhead. Return the way you came.

Alternate Approaches: Three trailheads provide reasonable access to this loop: Cave Creek from the northeast, Bronco from the southeast, and Spur Cross from the southwest. All make excellent hikes from any direction, though the general preference is to take the loop counterclockwise. Cottonwood is difficult either way, whereas Cave Creek is easier heading west and south.

Cave Creek is the shortest spur but guarantees an uphill return trip, and there are fewer camping options down near Spur Cross (which is for day use only). Bronco has the longest spur and is primarily for equestrians. Hikers from Bronco would want to camp near Matty's Fork.

DIRECTIONS: From the town of Cave Creek (north of Phoenix), take Spur Cross Road all the way north to where it terminates in the dirt lot that serves as parking for the county park. The dirt parking lot sees a lot of use. The trail store just down the road has some services. There are porta-potties just past the gate into the park, plus maps and other information. Entrance to the park requires a $3-per-person fee at the self-pay station. There is no fee indicated when returning from the national forest side.

Some Forest Service publications indicate that you can drive directly to the Skull Mesa trailhead in the national forest—this is not true. The road through Spur Cross is closed to private motor vehicles. Taking that road adds about 2.5 miles to the hike—each way.

GPS Trailhead Coordinates	19 COTTONWOOD 247/CAVE CREEK
UTM zone (WGS 84)	12S
Easting	412057.58
Northing	3750098.52
Latitude/Longitude	
North	33° 53'15.3"
West	111° 57' 03.7"

Four Peaks and Mazatzal Wilderness

4

Explore numerous high peaks, deep gorges, babbling river beds, near-silent deserts, hundred-year-old mining camps, or thousand-year-old Native American settlements

SCENERY: 🐾 🐾 🐾 🐾	DISTANCE: *9 miles*
TRAIL CONDITION: 🐾 🐾 🐾	HIKING TIME: *4.5 hours*
CHILDREN: 🐾 🐾	OUTSTANDING FEATURES: *Sweeping vistas of*
DIFFICULTY: 🐾 🐾 🐾	*(in order) Lake Roosevelt, Roosevelt Dam, the Salt*
SOLITUDE: 🐾 🐾 🐾	*River Canyon, and the Four Peaks range; crumbling*
	ruins; a reflector tower; Sonoran and transition eco-
	systems; and, in season, eagles and wildflowers

Vineyard Trail marches straight up the slopes from Roosevelt Lake, passing through two ecosystems and a scattering of history to provide outstanding vistas of both the Tonto Basin to the east and the Four Peaks range to the west. You'll climb past the work camp that was active when the dam was built and head to the abandoned signal tower, then follow the ridgeline past the old vineyard site for which the trail was named. This route is part of the Arizona Trail, which runs from Mexico to Utah.

🚶🚶 Vineyard Trail starts immediately southwest from the highway, heads around the wash, then ascends the next hill to reach an interpretive sign explaining that this was the site of the O'Rourke labor camp, built and occupied by the workers who built Roosevelt Dam. Indeed, if you bushwhack into the brush a bit, you may encounter an occasional foundation or remains of a retaining wall, but little else. Take the switchbacks up and through the "site." This starts a big climb.

Toward the top of the first hill, you'll notice how the road follows a trace jeep trail. That gray rock crunching beneath your feet was the roadbed originally used to haul equipment to the top of Vineyard Mountain. The road turns north by northwest, passing around Inspiration Point, and then continuing to climb west. The path levels out for a few hundred feet, coming north across the saddle between Inspiration Point and Vineyard Mountain, but then climbs Vineyard Mountain again. Look across the ravine, and notice the steeply

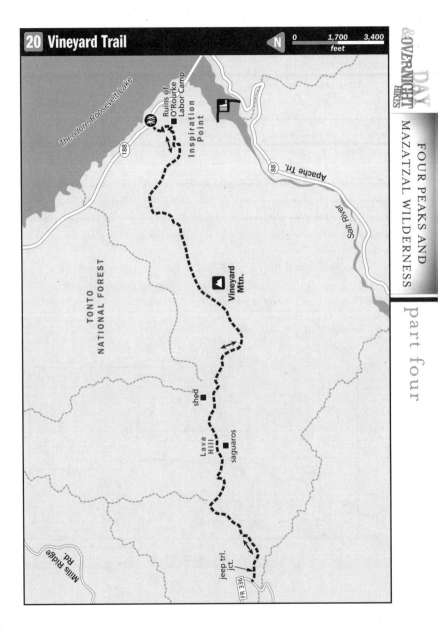

20 Vineyard Trail

N

0   1,700   3,400
feet

DAY
& OVERNIGHT
HIKES

FOUR PEAKS AND
MAZATZAL WILDERNESS

part four

Theodore Roosevelt Lake

Ruins of
O'Rourke
Labor Camp

Inspiration Point

188

Apache Trl.

88

Salt River

TONTO
NATIONAL FOREST

Vineyard Mtn.

shed

Lava
Hill

saguaros

jeep trl. jct.

FR 336

Mills Ridge Rd.

angled rock striations. That angle, formed when this whole range pushed up abruptly about 6 million years ago, matches the grade of your trail. That's why you're struggling.

After that second climb, the path levels briefly to switchback up the second part of Vineyard Mountain. If you face southeast while you catch your breath, you'll see Roosevelt Dam, a landmark construction of its day and still represented in Arizona's state seal.

Near the top of Vineyard Mountain, the rocks beneath your feet are now the color of burned brick. You've climbed 1,100 feet in about 1.5 miles. The trail goes near—but not to—the lonely reflector tower, which you can see to your left. If you're inclined, follow the remnants of the jeep trail to the base of the tower. But from there you'll see no more than what you see from the trail—a steel tower with a tan, metal square on top of it.

You've climbed into high desert chaparral: the tall grass and flowering weeds on this ridgeline are broken up by prickly pear, ocotillo, stunted Joshua trees, and smokethorn trees. On a good day, you might see bald eagles, which are making a comeback around the lake. If they were circling above you on this hike, they circle beside

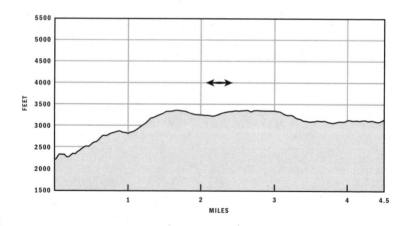

you now. Butterflies flutter in front of you. Keep an eye out for ant hills and the webs of trapdoor spiders underfoot—both are common on this trail. Follow the track as it winds northwest to skirt the mountain. To your right, you'll notice a large, corrugated-metal shed squatting lower on the ridge—this is all that remains of the vineyard that gives this trail its name.

As you leave the shed behind, the trail turns due west again to wind down a lava rock–covered hill. In spring, the slopes are also full-to-bursting with bright-yellow desert poppies. The narrow trail, a steep grade all the way down, is alternately overgrown with weeds or composed of nothing but lava rock. If you look down the slope, you'll see a stand of mildly obese saguaros dotting the slope. Beyond them, the wide Salt River flows through the canyon toward its next reservoir. On the other side of the water, you can see the graded dirt "highway" of Apache Trail.

Around the lava hill, the trail levels out to run along a wide ridge for the last mile. This is pleasant going, with packed dirt covering the trail most of the time. As you climb up the next hill, you'll pass a variety of (possibly mutant) cholla. Keep an eye out for the cactus wrens that nest in them.

Toward the top of the hill, you'll see Forest Road 336 ahead of you. Before you get there, the trail will merge with a barely visible remnant jeep trail for the last 200 yards or so. This signed junction (with AZT blazes and everything) is 4.45 miles from your start, and marks the official turnaround for this hike. Vineyard Trail continues along FR 336 south (left) through a wash then up a hill to a pullout. Vineyard Trail goes west another 2 miles from that point, heading through exactly this sort of countryside (only more uphill), until it terminates at FR 429 and the Mills Ridge trailhead. Arizona Trail continues on Four Peaks Trail 130, which starts at Mills Ridge.

If you still have gas, you could also follow FR 336 farther southwest about 1 mile to Buckhorn Spring, a lovely, tree-laden spot where the spring feeds Buckhorn Creek. You should know, though, that you'd drop 500 feet on the way down, which, of course, you'll have to climb back up. Return the way you came.

DIRECTIONS: From Phoenix, take AZ 87 (Beeline Highway) north to AZ 188. Follow AZ 188 east until just before the bridge near the dam. Alternately, you could take Apache Trail (AZ 88) from Mesa to AZ 188, then turn left (west) across this same bridge. You should know, though, that Apache Trail is a graded dirt road with many hairpin turns and an average speed limit of 25 mph. Park at the very first turnout on AZ 188 north of the bridge. Seriously, this is the first place you could possibly park a car. Cross AZ 188 and walk along the guardrail to the "Junction AZ 88½ mile" sign. Just beyond that sign is the marked trailhead for Vineyard Trail 131.

GPS Trailhead Coordinates	20 VINEYARD TRAIL
UTM zone (WGS 84)	12S
Easting	485073.3
Northing	3726302.6
Latitude/Longitude	
North	33° 40' 35.5"
West	111° 09' 39.7"

21 Four Peaks Loop

SCENERY: ✿ ✿ ✿ ✿
TRAIL CONDITION: ✿ ✿
CHILDREN: ✿
DIFFICULTY: ✿ ✿ ✿
SOLITUDE: ✿ ✿ ✿

DISTANCE: *11.4 miles*
HIKING TIME: *7 hours*
OUTSTANDING FEATURES: *Outstanding vistas of the Four Peaks and surrounding area, several different climate zones, a chance to see what your legs and lungs are made of*

This car-shuttle hike takes Oak Flat Trail straight up the slopes of the Four Peaks range to meet Four Peaks Trail in the wilderness area. Following this trail south along the slopes reveals a series of stunning vistas. The route then takes Chillicut Trail down the mountain and across some high chaparral to the Rock Creek trailhead. An easy car shuttle is required.

🚶🚶 The Oak Flat trailhead, not to be confused with the one in the Superstition Wilderness, is, indeed, surrounded by a number of large oak trees. Oak Flat Trail 123 starts due west from the sign. Follow the cairns across the creek and then start climbing the ridge. After a couple of switchbacks, the trail goes straight up through the manzanitas, scrub oak, and beargrass. There are few trees, and none near the trail—nothing between the sun and the gravel path but you.

To your left, Brown's Peak, the tallest and most northern of the Four Peaks, glowers down at you. To your right, you can see FR 445 winding up the canyon to the trailhead, and beyond it, Roosevelt Lake stretches out to fill the Tonto Basin with this year's collected snow run-off. Soon, you turn south to start climbing and climbing and climbing.

The gravel trench heads roughly southwest. The unrelenting climb (1,700 feet in 1.7 miles) may cause you to doubt the overall recreational nature of this pursuit. When you pass the rain gauge, which looks like a sideways windmill, you're about two thirds done. Oaks and pines shade small patches of the trail.

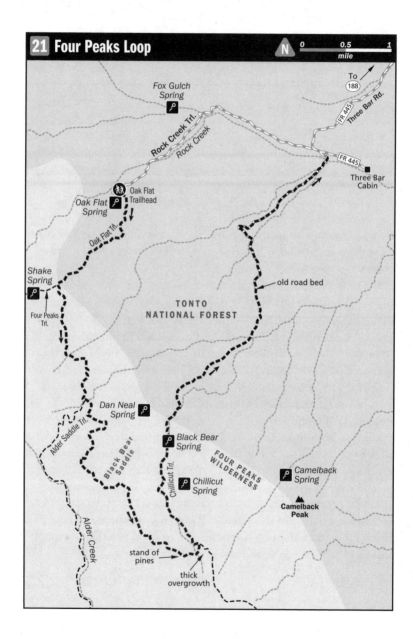

N

0   0.5   1
mile

To
188

Three Bar Rd.

FR 445

Fox Gulch
Spring

Rock Creek Trl.

Rock Creek

FR 445

Three Bar
Cabin

Oak Flat
Trailhead

Oak Flat
Spring

Oak Flat Trl.

old road bed

Shake
Spring

Four Peaks
Trl.

TONTO
NATIONAL FOREST

Dan Neal
Spring

Alder Saddle Trl.

Black
Bear
Saddle

Black Bear
Spring

Chillicut Trl.

Chillicut
Spring

FOUR PEAKS
WILDERNESS

Camelback
Spring

Camelback
Peak

Alder Creek

stand of
pines

thick
overgrowth

The little sign announcing the wilderness boundary is your "almost there" mark. Shortly thereafter, the trail reaches a T-intersection with Four Peaks Trail 130. The sign might be confusing; turn left. Four Peaks Trail goes due south, climbing another 500 feet to level out at around the 5,800-foot line. The brown basalt glistens with pyrite, while towering ponderosa pine trees poke above the abundant scrub bushes.

At the top of the climb, the trail winds southwest. There are a few ups and downs, but overall, the trail stays at the 5,800-foot line, with just enough hazard to keep you from getting lost in the vistas.

At 3.3 miles, you cross a creek and come to the signed junction with Alder Saddle Trail. Alder Saddle is a steep climb to its namesake, where it dead-ends. Stay on Four Peaks Trail. As you wind around the slopes heading toward Buckhorn Mountain (that high point to the south) every view to your right (west) of the Four Peaks will be more stunning than the last. Ration camera memory accordingly.

At 4.5 miles, you cross Black Bear Saddle, near springs of the same name. The fence line you might see on top of the ridgeline above you separates Gila County (east) from Maricopa County (west).

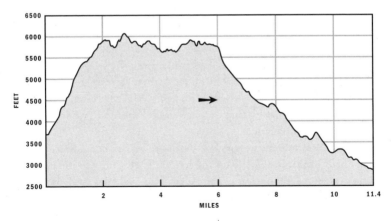

Past this saddle, you encounter the first bit of real trail treachery as bushes conspire to shove you down the slope. If you take your time and plan your steps, their schemes will surely fail.

A mile later, a stand of pine and oak shade the trail, growing upslope amid granite boulders. Past the stand of pines, you hit real overgrowth. Yes, the trail goes through those bushes. Really. Seep willow bush chokes off all but the bottom two feet of the trail, obliging any creatures taller than a rabbit to push their way through the thick shrubbery. Where you don't step on plants—that's the trail. After a couple hundred yards, though, you plow through the worst of it. Soon after, you come to the signed intersection with Chillicut Trail 132.

Some maps and descriptions depict this trail as ending well downslope of this junction, but recent maintenance has allowed it to climb all the way up to the Four Peaks route. These same sources show Four Peaks Trail going straight over the top of Buckhorn Mountain, but it now winds around the east slope. From your perspective, though, you simply take the left turn to head northwest and downhill.

Chillicut Trail does not mess around, dropping 500 feet in less than 0.5 miles before entering the ravine near Chillicut Spring. This well-cairned route winds through the underbrush and beneath the blackened skeletons of once-towering oak trees, many of which are spectacular even in death. Past the springs, you follow the streambed. Oaks and sycamore line the babbling creek, and your passage will disperse a cloud of butterflies. The route down the stream is easy to find, but fairly rugged. Take your time and watch your step. As you descend farther, you travel an easy dirt singletrack through transition scrubland. Crisscrossing the drainage several times will often require a little bit of bouldering.

About 1 mile past the springs, before the creek bends east, you switchback out of the ravine on the left bank, climbing to the higher and drier chaparral on top of the ridge. The trail goes straight down the ridgeline to the confluence of creeks that marks the start of Baldy Canyon.

Cross the creek to the left. Past this, the trail heads due north, up and over the next ridge. The trail past this is a remnant jeep trail, bouncing through increasingly lower chaparral. It continues north, down and then up a ravine, and then turns east to follow the ridge finger down the last mile. The last 0.25 miles follows the creek bed to its confluence with Rock Creek. Across Rock Creek is the trailhead.

DIRECTIONS: From the Phoenix area, take AZ 87 north until its junction with AZ 188, which you'll take south (a right turn) toward Lake Roosevelt. Ten miles south of Pumpkin Center (the only town you'll pass), look for Three Bar Road (a.k.a. Forest Road 445—though the sign on the highway says "Three Bar") to your right. Follow the graded dirt road about 3.5 miles, until it forks. A short distance down the left (southeast) branch, you will find the Rock Creek trailhead. Another 2.5 miles up the right (northwest) branch, you come to the Oak Flat trailhead. Getting to Oak Flat requires a high-clearance vehicle.

GPS Trailhead Coordinates	21 FOUR PEAKS LOOP
	OAK FLAT
UTM zone (WGS 84)	12S
Easting	472130.22
Northing	3729235.18
Latitude/Longitude	
North	33° 42' 9.78"
West	111° 18' 2.69"

GPS Trailhead Coordinates	ROCK CREEK
UTM zone (WGS 84)	12S
Easting	475328.27
Northing	3732699.84
Latitude/Longitude	
North	33° 44' 2.56"
West	111° 15' 58.8"

SCENERY: ✿ ✿ ✿	DISTANCE: *8.6 miles*
TRAIL CONDITION: ✿ ✿	HIKING TIME: *12 hours (2 days)*
CHILDREN: ✿ ✿ ✿	OUTSTANDING FEATURES: *Dramatic vistas,*
DIFFICULTY: ✿ ✿ ✿	*wildlife, the death and life of forests after fire*
SOLITUDE: ✿ ✿ ✿ ✿	

*This hike follows the southernmost leg of Mazatzal Divide Trail, which roughly fol-
lows the top of the range that separates the Verde River drainages from the Salt River
drainages. The first part of this hike, up, around, and then just past Mount Peeley,
can be done as a moderate day hike. The second part, walking along the ridgeline roughly north to Bear Springs Saddle, would be an easy overnight, except for trail
conditions that make for a moderate hike, with stretches of "you've-got-to-be-
kidding." This hike, along with the rest of Divide Trail, is part of Arizona Trail
(AZT), which runs from Mexico to Utah.*

From the trailhead, take Cornucopia Trail 86, which follows the old roadbed 0.5 miles toward Mount Peeley through pine
and juniper woodlands. At this point, you come to the signed junction with Matzatzal Divide Trail 23. Go right (up) to start climbing
the big, well-defined switchbacks that ascend the slopes of Mount
Peeley, taking you up more than 900 feet in about 1 mile. The grade
is gentle; it is the lung-crunching elevation that provides most of the
challenge.

The Precambrian rock that forms the southern Mazatzal range
exposes itself as dark, flaky shale toward the bottom of the mountains
but as brighter, copper-colored quartzite toward the top. Manzanita,
scrub oak, and some yucca provide the flora, so you won't have much
shade as you mount switchback after switchback. The word "mazatzal" is supposed to be an Aztec word meaning "land of many deer."

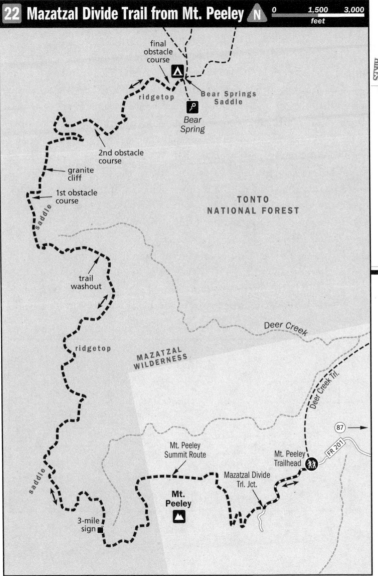

22 Mazatzal Divide Trail from Mt. Peeley

N

0   1,500   3,000
              feet

final obstacle course

ridgetop

Bear Springs Saddle

Bear Spring

2nd obstacle course

granite cliff

1st obstacle course

saddle

TONTO NATIONAL FOREST

trail washout

ridgetop

Deer Creek

MAZATZAL WILDERNESS

Deer Creek Trl.

saddle

Mt. Peeley Summit Route

Mt. Peeley Trailhead

87

FR 201

Mazatzal Divide Trl. Jct.

Mt. Peeley

3-mile sign

This area is far north of anywhere the Aztecs ever controlled, but the Hohokam, who settled widely in this area until about the 1500s, traded as far south as the Aztec Empire.

There are certainly deer about, but they have a lot of country to hide in. Smaller critters, ladybugs, and butterflies abound.

At 1.5 miles, a rock cairn indicates the route to the 7,034-foot summit of Mount Peeley, an unmarked route straight up the forested slopes. You're on your own with that. Wind around the north slope of the mountain through pine, juniper, and oak forest. This area is untouched by fire, and well shaded. Go 180 degrees around the slopes before continuing west around the ravine to the next ridge.

At 3.4 miles you find the toppled remains of the 3-mile marker (probably 3 miles from what is now the Cornucopia junction). At 4.4 miles you come to a saddle. Only a few oak grow here, allowing a good view off of both sides. To your right (north), the whole Deer Creek drainage drops into Maple Draw, then farther, to Bar Canyon, and eventually to Lake Roosevelt. To your left (south) the whole Lower Verde Basin opens up. Horseshoe Lake spreads out in front of the New River Mountains. And beyond that, those thin blue peaks

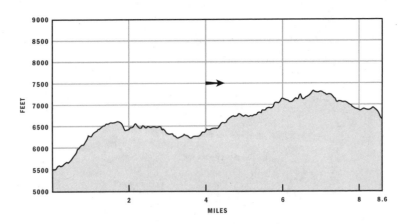

are the Bradshaw Mountains south of Prescott. This is the turn-around for the easy day hike.

Past here, the trail follows the ridgeline north. Divide Trail does a lot of winding, being originally a horse trail, where level grades are best. Given that, and the nature of ridgelines, you can take an awful lot of steps and still seem not to have gone very far. For example, from here you can still make out the trailhead. Bear Springs Saddle would be only 2.5 miles from the trailhead if you were one of the hawks that circles occasionally overhead.

The trees give way to manzanita bushes lining the trail and the rest of the ridgetop. Most of these are young, and while they crowd the trail, they do not block it. After about 5 miles, you cross a saddle and suddenly find you must pick your way along a thin trail along a grass-covered slope. After about 6 miles, you turn a corner westward around the ridgeline to find yourself back in pine forest.

But the trail maintenance (mostly done by volunteers, by the way) you have been enjoying ends here. And soon, at 6.4 miles, you find the trail washed away completely as it crosses a pair of sizable washes. Climb upslope through the scree to pick your way across and then down through the brush.

Up to now charred trees have been rare, but they will become more common as you continue. In 0.5 miles you cross a high saddle (just shy of 7,000 feet) and enter the burn zone proper. The saddle's western slope is a wilderness of charred trees. Nothing green grows higher than your knees, when there's any green at all. Take a break here, because the rest of the way will be tough going.

In 2004 the lightning-sparked Willow Fire burned nearly 120,000 acres, much of it in this wilderness. You enter now one of the southern reaches of that disaster area. Fire is part of the cycle of these forests, but it still take decades for a burned area to return to anything like normal. Meanwhile, tall, charred stumps stick out, or fall across bare and rapidly eroding gravel. Shrubbery will contain this erosion in a few years (it has already started to encroach the trail), but recent rains have washed much of a once-broad trail down the hillside.

The trail heads left, around the western slope of this next hill. Follow the orange ribbons; they may be your only guide in many places. The next 0.25 miles will be a military-level obstacle course as you follow the steep, slippery goat trail over and around a series of charred, fallen logs and other obstructions. You will get sooty. Then the trail improves, relatively, though you still push through the Gambel oak saplings that crowd it. Decades from now, the stronger ones will have starved the weaker ones from above and below to tower over whatever becomes of this trail. Meanwhile, though, they're in the way. More troublesome is the gooseberry (or some relative thereof), often crouching within the micro-stands of oak, waiting to shred a limb or pack with their raptor-like thorns.

You pass a large formation of granite before topping the next ridge and turning eastward. In less than 0.5 miles you turn abruptly westward; a move you might miss if you don't keep an eye out for orange ribbons. In another couple thousand feet, the trail bends around again, passing between a pair of boulders as it does so. From this spot, the whole western Mazatzal range opens up to your left. The trail winds to your right and begins a second obstacle course, with a more even grade but even more fallen logs. Below, you can see clearly where the fire blazed up drainages, leaving a wide trail of naked stumps.

The trail then climbs back to the top of the ridge and follows a manzanita-covered finger northeast for a short while. It will, and you have to watch for it, break to the left before climbing up through the sapling manzanitas toward the bluff-top crowned with a stand of surviving pines. Honestly, if you miss that turn, bushwhacking over the top of the ridge is no harder than taking the trail, for you will encounter the third and final obstacle course as the trail turns east then south, following the slope of the ridge.

But then it switchbacks one more time to drop you on top of Bear Springs Saddle. This pleasant stand of pine and oak was, by some fortune, spared the torch. A few good campsites can be found, with a bed of pine needles to cushion your bed and—ahem—plenty of firewood. You will also find the cairned spur trail to Bear Springs perpendicular to the saddle to your right.

The 0.8-mile spur trail is every bit as rough as the one that got you here. It dead-ends at the fern-covered gulley that contains the springs, where there is a concrete basin, at least a yard deep, filled with green, slimy water. This is one of the few reliable water sources along this route, but clearly you'll want to filter it.

Mazatzal Divide Trail goes much farther, all the way to City Trailhead, 27 miles in total. Before the fire, it was common to camp on the next saddle north, but that saddle hasn't fared as well as this one has.

In the morning, return the way you came.

DIRECTIONS: From Fountain Hills, head north on AZ 87 about 40 miles to the signed Sycamore Creek (FR 627) turnoff just north of milepost 222. At the T-intersection, turn right (north) onto FR 201. At the fork with FR 25, about 1 mile later, stay right to stay on 201. Drive about 8 miles along 201, heading over and around numerous ridgelines. The road dead-ends at the trailhead—a bare lot with no services.

FR 201 supposedly requires 4WD, but if it's dry, it is certainly passable in any high- to medium-clearance vehicle. A regular passenger car might also work, but that would test your nerves. If the road is wet, you definitely need a 4WD.

GPS Trailhead Coordinates	22 MAZATZAL DIVIDE TRAIL FROM MOUNT PEELEY
UTM zone (WGS 84)	12S
Easting	456542.79
Northing	3762884.1
Latitude/Longitude	
North	34° 00' 20.4"
West	111° 28' 14.2"

SCENERY: ☘ ☘ ☘	DISTANCE: *23.2 miles*
TRAIL CONDITION: ☘ ☘	HIKING TIME: *13 hours (2 days)*
CHILDREN: ☘	OUTSTANDING FEATURES: *Wildlife, isola-*
DIFFICULTY: ☘ ☘ ☘	*tion, scenic overlooks of several canyons, choice of*
SOLITUDE: ☘ ☘ ☘ ☘	*two riverbanks to camp at*

This hike follows the northern third of Verde River Trail down the well-named Hardscrabble Mesa and into the Mazatzal Wilderness. It then follows Road Mesa down, crosses a drainage, and climbs up and over Cedar Bench before finally descending toward the Verde River near its confluence with Fossil Creek. A mile from the river, the trail forks, giving a near-even choice of camping on the banks of the Verde River or those of Fossil Creek. Don't be fooled by the latitude; this is a very tough hike in the summer heat.

🚶🚶 From the vehicle barrier at the trailhead, the crumbling jeep trail wanders south, through juniper-studded grasslands, slowly descending the buttes. For much of the way, the roadbed is so choked with lava rocks as to offer no advantage (other than navigational) over simply bushwhacking across the ancient lava flow.

Ahead, you can see the Mazatzal range to the south, and the top of the Verde Canyon to the southwest. In about 1 mile, the trail starts winding a little more to the southwest and becomes a little more recognizable as a road, though you will not mistake it for an easy means of conveyance. It remains simply the least overgrown stretch of lava rock.

The short juniper trees break up the monotony of the turquoise-colored grass and prickly pear but offer precious little shade. Between the rocks, the soil sports cracks wide enough to support spider webs and deep enough to eat hiking sticks. Yet the grade

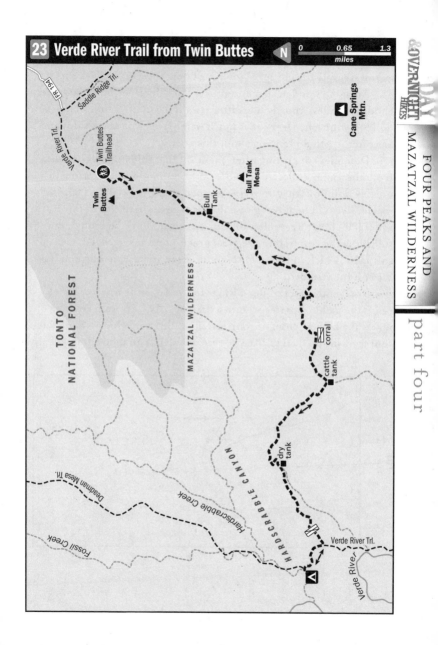

23 Verde River Trail from Twin Buttes

N

0   0.65   1.3
miles

Cane Springs Mtn.

FR 194

Saddle Ridge Trl.

Verde River Trl.

Twin Buttes Trailhead

Twin Buttes

Bull Tank Mesa

Bull Tank

MAZATZAL WILDERNESS

TONTO NATIONAL FOREST

corral

cattle tank

dry tank

Deadman Mesa Trl.

Fossil Creek

Hardscrabble Creek

HARDSCRABBLE CANYON

Verde River Trl.

Verde River

is barely perceptible, though you are descending from the trailhead elevation of almost 5,900 feet. In fact, you'll barely notice the grade as you struggle to find space for your boots between the lava rocks.

An aging wooden sign announces the wilderness boundary after about 1.5 miles. Shortly thereafter, you'll pass Bull Tank, a large cow tank, to your left. Deer get as much water from this as cows do, and are often spotted prancing about this area.

Defenders of grazing often mention that wild animals benefit from the waters collected in cattle tanks. Opponents of grazing just as quickly point out that the water trapped in the tanks didn't appear by magic; it would be flowing or collecting somewhere else in the drainage if left alone. Regardless of your position, don't be fooled into following the cow trail to the great green pond surrounded by deep soft mud, which indisputably benefits algae and a wide range of bugs. Stay on the roadbed.

You gently descend Road Ridge to the 4.5-mile mark, at which point the path drops steeply into a drainage. The dry wash crossing marks the halfway point of your march to the river, which is a reliable source of shade, if an unlikely source of water. You then climb steeply

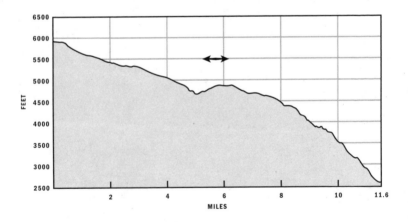

out of the ravine on your way to the top of Cedar Bench, turning to the west as you go. Once you're actually on top of the Bench, the rock cover eases a bit. The trail is not smooth by any stretch, but you tread on dirt here and there for as much as a hundred yards at a time.

A mile past the wash, you'll see a barbed-wire gate, a corral, and other cowboy artifacts to your left. The trail going through this gate is tempting but leads to a dead end. Stay straight (west), following the cairns down the old road and farther into the juniper.

Just past 6 miles, the road becomes a heavily eroded, rubble-filled wash, making travel difficult as you descend off the Bench. In 0.5 miles, you pass another cattle tank. Past the tank, there is a 0.25-mile section where the grass has grown into the roadway such that the slope is essentially trackless. You must lurch cairn to cairn through the grass and lava rock as the route turns somewhat north. The good news is that the road reappears after 0.25 miles. The bad news is that it appears as another rock-filled wash as it steeply drops.

It soon levels out, meaning it reverts to the regular, gradual grade. At about 8 miles, Verde Trail starts winding around the side of the ridge, over the top, and then down the ridgeline. Along here, you will be able to see various perspectives of the Verde Canyon opening up before you, in addition to the gorge of Hell's Hole (not to be confused with the one in the Salome Wilderness—a whole separate hike). The roadbed switchbacking down these ridges is a wide, orange dirt track filled with gray lava rock. As you cross the second ridgetop and continue down past a dry cattle tank, you start seeing yucca and barrel cacti as the ecology shifts to chaparral.

The trail thins considerably as you pick your way down the ridge into the canyon. Cairns guide you through the tall grass between the prickly pear. It is slow going down this steep and rocky slope because there are precious few places to put your feet. This awful stretch lasts about 0.25 miles before the roadbed levels out both horizontally and vertically, and you begin to see isolated stretches of bare dirt again.

Somewhere around here, you'll want to stop and take some pictures of the Verde Canyon as it stretches down to the south. That's where you, and what's left of your boots, will be going.

At 9 miles, you cross the ridgetop, and then a singletrack splits off from the roadway to lead you around the ridge, down toward the river. Past this point, you will be traveling on a relatively normal trail. You will notice, however, that the grade becomes steeper (if not on the way in, then certainly on the way out). You have passed into chaparral at this point, with more prickly pear, scrub oak, and our old friend the catclaw coming to greet you trailside. At 9.7 miles, halfway down your final descent, you must open (and close) a gate. You've dropped to 3,300 feet at this spot, and the river can be seen below.

Soon after, at the top of the last little hill, you find a wooden sign held in place by rocks next to its broken post. It tells you that you are 9 miles from the Twin Buttes trailhead (which is a bit optimistic) and 1.25 miles from the river (which is about right). The packed dirt continues to the left of the sign. To the right, however, is an alternate trail, marked only by cairns, that takes you to Fossil Creek, upstream of the confluence on the other side of this ridge.

Both trails from this point are within 0.1 mile and 100 feet of elevation of each other. The route profiled goes to Fossil Creek, which has clearer water, more shade, and a better selection of campsites. However, there are plenty of places to plop your bag on the wide banks of the Verde.

To your right is a spur of what is properly designated Deadman Mesa Trail 17. Descending westward toward the creek, it is part remnant road and part cairn-to-cairn bushwhack across the burr-infested brush—dropping 500 feet in just more than 0.5 miles. You pass among mesquite trees before entering the lush, riparian corridor of the creek bed.

For a hundred years, Fossil Creek had seen a fraction of its normal flow, as much of its water was diverted to a pair of small hydroelectric power plants. These plants have been decommissioned and are in the process of being removed in a wondrous, cooperative effort of the utility company, environmental groups, and various government agencies. The result quadrupled the creek's flow literally overnight.

Consequently, the lower banks of Fossil Creek are choked with huge piles of driftwood and other debris that washed down in the gush of freedom, piling up between the cottonwoods and sycamores like the nests of monstrous, sloppy birds. The clear, mineral-heavy waters of the creek flow merrily in and around this convoluted tangle, forming numerous little pools and falls before finally emptying into the wide, silt-laden Verde River. Deadman Mesa Trail follows the creek upstream (north) until it climbs the rocky face of its namesake to meet Forest Road 591, some 4.5 miles away.

To the south, on the other side of the butte, Verde River Trail continues past the sign as a steep, packed-dirt track winding down the canyon toward the green river below. You reach the bank on the south end of a bend that originates just below the Fossil Creek confluence. Again, you drop 600 feet in just under 1 mile and traverse a stand of mesquite trees before reaching the cottonwood saplings that line the boulder-strewn banks.

The Verde (Spanish for "green") River has been designated Wild and Scenic along where its course defines the western boundary of the Mazatzal Wilderness (the Wild and Scenic designation and the wilderness boundary are coincidental). The steep walls on the far bank leave this trail as the only practical land access to this stretch of the river. Verde River Trail continues another 17 miles, following the river for much of that journey, until it terminates at the Sheep's Bridge trailhead in the southwest corner of the wilderness, just before the river flows into Horseshoe Reservoir.

Wherever you camp, make certain to top off your water before the journey back up. Both the Verde and Fossil Creek flow through

cattle country, and their water should be treated before drinking.
Return the way you came.

DIRECTIONS: From Payson, take AZ 87 north about 17 miles,
through Pine to the town of Strawberry. In Strawberry, turn left at
the Strawberry Lodge to follow Fossil Creek Road west through town.
Just after the pavement ends, look for a turnoff to the left for FR
428 (a more prominent sign advertises a retreat). In just more than
0.5 miles, turn right down FR 194 and follow that road 5 bumpy
miles until you start circling a ranch. High-clearance vehicles are
recommended, and a 4WD might be necessary for the last 0.25
miles as you climb a hill past the line house. You could park lesser
vehicles on the pullout at the base of the hill. The trailhead has a
fire pit but no services.

GPS Trailhead Coordinates	23 VERDE RIVER TRAIL FROM TWIN BUTTES
UTM zone (WGS 84)	12S
Easting	447253.2
Northing	3800999.39
Latitude/Longitude	
North	34° 20' 56.3"
West	111° 34' 24.7"

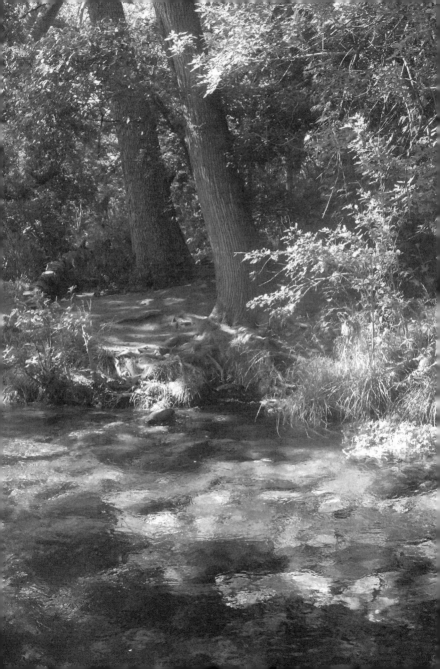

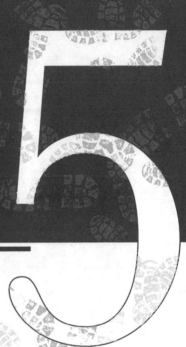

The Central
Mountains

5

Explore
numerous
high peaks
deep gorges
babbling
river
beds
near-silen
deserts,
hundred-
year-old
mining
camps,
or thousand-
year-old
Native
American
settlements

SCENERY: ✿ ✿	DISTANCE: *5.8 miles*
TRAIL CONDITION: ✿ ✿ ✿	HIKING TIME: *3 hours*
CHILDREN: ✿ ✿ ✿ ✿	OUTSTANDING FEATURES: *Views of Pleasant*
DIFFICULTY: ✿	*Valley and Hell's Gate Wilderness, cowboy ruins*
SOLITUDE: ✿ ✿ ✿	

This easy hike crosses Tonto Creek, following Bear Flats Trail over a couple of hills. It then splits off to travel along Mescal Ridge in the eastern end of the Hell's Gate Wilderness Area. Along the way, it provides splendid views of the Mogollon Rim, Pleasant Valley, and the canyons of the Hell's Gate Wilderness. This little-known route is still easy to follow and provides a quick scenic hike without the crowds found across the highway on the Rim.

🚶🚶 Head toward the bridge and cross Tonto Creek near the sign. Tonto Creek is perennial—if the water is high, this may be the hardest part of the hike.

Look for the sign on the far side indicating Bear Flats PV Trail 178 (PV = Pleasant Valley). This also indicates it's 0.5 miles to Mescal Ridge Trail. In fact, it's closer to 1 mile and mostly uphill. The trail follows near the creek until you come to a gate, which you'll have to open and close. Go right, following the singletrack. Soon, that singletrack will cut steeply up the pine-covered ridge. Do not follow the angler trails that continue along the creek. You want to take the steepest trail up the hill. The path joins the old roadway halfway to the hilltop, where you find a sign announcing the wilderness boundary.

The old roadway, which doubles as the trail, hooks around to the left. Several fallen logs block it as it drops into and across a ravine heading east. Past the big stump near the creek bed, the old roadway goes straight up the next hill, gaining close to 400 feet in 0.25 miles. The old jeep trail here has been reduced to a wide trench filled

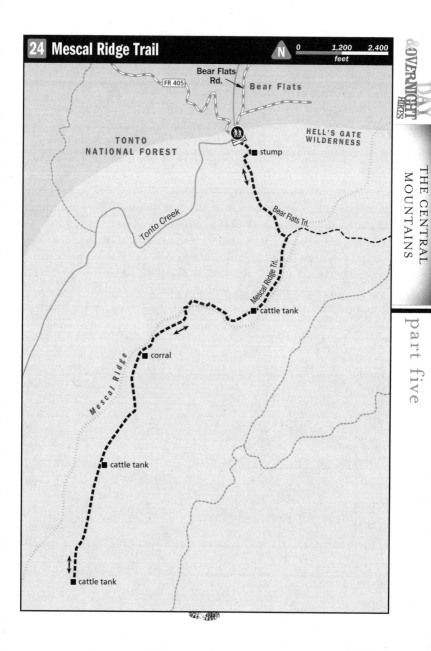

24 Mescal Ridge Trail

N

0   1,200   2,400
feet

Bear Flats Rd.

Bear Flats

HELL'S GATE WILDERNESS

TONTO NATIONAL FOREST

FR 405

stump

Bear Flats Trl.

Tonto Creek

Mescal Ridge Trl.

cattle tank

corral

Mescal Ridge

cattle tank

cattle tank

with orange stumble-rocks winding up through the pines and oak. Toward the top, the trail winds southward, becoming a singletrack through the manzanita scrub as it goes. Behind you, to the north, the Mogollon Rim stretches unevenly across the horizon.

At 0.75 miles, you come to the signed T-junction with Mescal Ridge Trail 186. Take the right, down Mescal Ridge Trail. Bear Flats Trail continues several more miles southeast, winding down toward Haigler Canyon. The orange singletrack of Mescal Ridge Trail winds up and along the ridgetop. Hawks may circle overhead. Alligator juniper, manzanita bushes, various species of yucca, and a smattering of prickly pear line the route. To your east, you will have fine views of Horse Mountain and south of that, Pleasant Valley.

The native people have used the various species of agave or yucca plants to provide food, clothing, intoxicants, and many other necessities. The word "mescal" generally refers to any liquor (other than tequila) distilled from the agave plant. Most of the species of agave found in the Tonto can be seen somewhere on this hike: the towering candelabras of the century plants, the thin-bladed sotol, and, of course, the yucca itself.

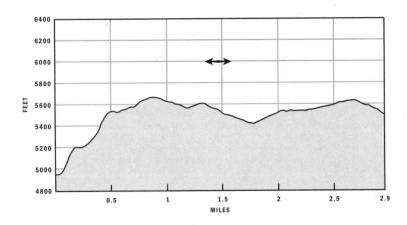

Despite the popularity of Bear Flats, this trail is lightly used. You may be breaking spider webs along your way. On the trail, you may see deer scat and the like, but the cow pies indicate why this trail was blazed in the first place.

Overgrazing by cattle decimates not only the normal cover of grasses and shrubs but all the species that depend on them, from native deer and elk, which forage the same flora, to turkey, quail, rodents, and lizards, which depend upon the groundcover for survival. Most rangelands in the western United States have been overgrazed.

The 26,000 cattle grazing the Tonto, or more specifically, the excrement they leave behind, has also made every river in the Tonto unpotable without treatment. Drought has forced the Forest Service to cut grazing to 20 percent of maximum allotments over the past years, but it's still not hard to spot the damage. On the other hand, without grazing, this trail, and many like it, would likely not be here at all.

As you cross the first hill on the ridgeline, keep an eye out to your right for a small cattle tank. Frequently dry, it usually presents itself as a crater of mud surrounded by manzanitas.

At 1.5 miles the trail starts a brief but rocky descent into a little saddle between hills. Down in this saddle you find a stock corral, in poor but marginally serviceable condition. A lonely little cholla cactus grows in the center of the corral. Past the corral the trail climbs a second ridge. The prickly pear, along with the rest of the scrub forest, closes in on the rocky trail through here. Then you arrive at a cattle tank: a 25-foot wide, stagnant pond of water surrounded by green grass and determined mosquitoes. As you move on past the tank, you'll see more vistas of the pastures of Pleasant Valley through the stunted trees.

The Pleasant Valley wars, which provided gainful employment to Billy the Kid and a small army of similar gunslingers, were part of the process by which cowboys "settled" the West. They shot at each other, of course, over grazing rights. Where the movies depict desert shootouts, most, in fact, took place in grassy juniper scrubland such as you walk through now.

In another 0.5 miles you encounter a third cattle tank, slightly smaller than the one you just passed. A barbed-wire fence surrounds the tank, but there is an opening to your right if you want a closer look at the brackish pond.

Neither trail following the outer fence goes anywhere. Return the way you came.

DIRECTIONS: From Payson, follow AZ 260 east 11 miles, passing the Ponderosa Campground. Look right for the turnoff to FR 405, which leads to Bear Flats. Follow the graded dirt road for 3.2 miles, winding over a couple of ridges to the trailhead just south of the bridge. Across the bridge is private land. The trailhead has some campsites but no services.

GPS Trailhead Coordinates	24 MESCAL RIDGE TRAIL
UTM zone (WGS 84)	12S
Easting	493723.4
Northing	3793642
Latitude/Longitude	
North	34° 17' 02.2"
West	111° 04' 05.5"

25 Pinal Mountain Loop

SCENERY: ✿ ✿ ✿ ✿	DISTANCE: *10.4 miles*
TRAIL CONDITION: ✿ ✿ ✿	HIKING TIME: *5.5 hours*
CHILDREN: ✿ ✿ ✿	OUTSTANDING FEATURES: *Scenic vistas,*
DIFFICULTY: ✿ ✿ ✿	*cowboy ruins, manzanita trees, mixed conifer forest*
SOLITUDE: ✿ ✿ ✿ ✿	

This loop hits some of the better parts of the Pinal Mountain system of trails. Starting from the Icehouse CCC Recreation Area, it follows Telephone Trail up Telephone Ridge, dipping briefly into Icehouse Canyon to pass by a spring, then climbing back up the ridge before descending into Six Shooter Canyon. There, near an old sawmill site and a flowing creek, it meets Six Shooter Trail, which will take you back down through lush forest, then transition scrub, and finally the chaparral back to Icehouse CCC.

🏃 Find the wooden Telephone Trail 192 sign on the northwest side of the outhouse. (You'll return to Six Shooter Trailhead, 200 feet away on the southeast side of the outhouse.) This trail heads northwest, quickly crossing the road. Soon after, it reaches a signed fork with Icehouse Trail 198. Go left (basically south) along Telephone Trail.

Start your climb up Telephone Ridge through thick chaparral consisting mostly of manzanita, scrub oak, and sugarberry. Soon the climb becomes steep and the scrub around you affords little shade. At about 1 mile in and around the 5,000-foot line, the trail starts switchbacking a little; juniper and, later, pine shade your path on occasion. Behind you, you can see the trailhead, and far beyond it, the Globe/Miami area and the monumental copper-mining operations where monstrous vehicles busily reduce whole mountains into piles of gravel.

As you wind through the thin pine forest, you'll have to cross numerous fallen logs and open and close three gates. After the third

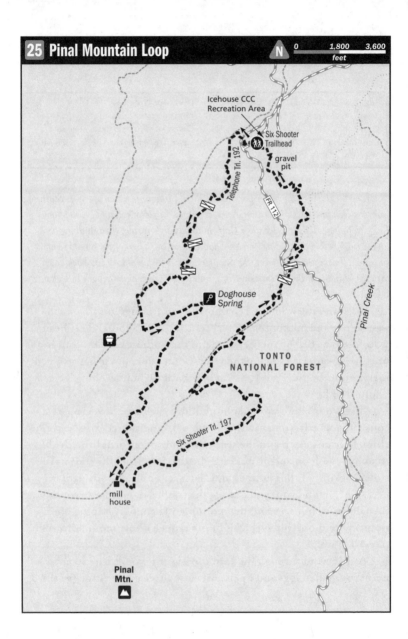

N

0   1,800   3,600
feet

Icehouse CCC
Recreation Area

Six Shooter
Trailhead

gravel
pit

Telephone Trl. 192

FR 112

Doghouse
Spring

TONTO
NATIONAL FOREST

Pinal Creek

Six Shooter Trl. 197

mill
house

Pinal
Mtn.

gate, the trail bends southwest into Icehouse Canyon, where it will re-merge with Icehouse Trail near Doghouse Spring. This spring reliably spills water across the trail through the little creek. Old cowboy relics lie among the sycamores, walnuts, and big pine trees. Plenty of logs provide shady resting places. At 5,800 feet, you've already gained 1,200 feet from the trailhead.

Telephone and Icehouse share the same dirt for 200 feet, before they split. Icehouse continues due south as a remnant road, while Telephone climbs the ridge as a singletrack, heading more southeast. Take that left, up the ridge to climb steeply out of the pine and then turn east into the manzanita-dominated chaparral that covers the ridgetop. The manzanita can grow quite tall through here, more of a small tree than the large bush it usually forms. On occasion, it will seem like you're passing through a tunnel of iron-colored shrubs.

At the ridgetop, the trail bends sharply back to the south to climb the ridgeline toward Pinal Mountain. Telephone Ridge was once, as the name implies, the route by which telephone and other utility lines were run up the mountain. These are all underground now, but the maintenance route remains as this trail.

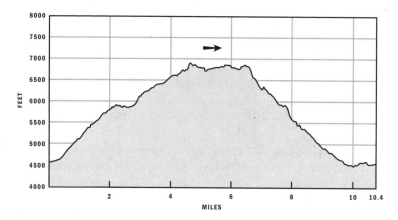

At around 4.5 miles, you start winding down into Six Shooter Canyon, where the manzanita yields to tall pines. Just past the 5-mile mark, keep an eye out for the old sawmill site to your right. Not much remains of the circa-1900 sawmill or the cabin site beyond— just flat ground and scraps of metal siding rusting in the woods. Just beyond this, you will cross Six Shooter Creek, surrounded by big riparian trees such as Fremont cottonwood, Arizona sycamore, and hackberry trees. You won't encounter a finer spot for lunch.

A hundred yards beyond the creek, Telephone Trail terminates in a T-intersection with Six Shooter Trail 197. To your right (south), the Six Shooter climbs one more steep mile to its southern origin at the Ferndell trailhead near the mountaintop. To the left, it descends the ridge to the north. Go left, watching right for a mineshaft-turned-spring just off the trail within the first 100 yards.

The first part of Six Shooter is an old roadway hovering at around the 6,800-foot line, but it soon becomes a singletrack as it descends through marvelous mixed-conifer forest. Gambel oaks and various pine and spruce dominate above, while all manner of bushes and weeds crowd the roadbed below. This area is a known and popular habitat for deer, ring-tailed cats, and mountain bikers.

As the trail turns west to switchback down the ridge into Six Shooter Canyon, the forest thins out into a more common mix of pine and oak. You cross Six Shooter Creek as it tumbles down through a mishmash of granite and basalt, cottonwood and hackberry. The trail roughly follows the creek north and down, crossing it several times, as the pine forest is replaced by oak and juniper scrub. Just shy of 9 miles, you pass through a gate, and then cross Forest Road 112.

You could follow the forest road left (northwest) to go back to the trailhead, and no one would fault you for that. Such a route would be easier in several ways. Six Shooter Trail, though, crosses the road to continue another 1.5 miles through the manzanita-covered hills.

Just beyond the road, you make a rough and rocky wash crossing—the dry remains of Six Shooter Creek. Past this, the trail becomes a rock-filled old jeep trail until it reaches the intersection with Check Dam Trail 190, which continues south. Six Shooter, though, splits off west as a singletrack, passing through an old gravel quarry marked with a scattering of quartz and then emerging at the east end of Icehouse CCC trailhead.

DIRECTIONS: On US 60 east traveling through Globe, exit either left on Broad Street, traveling through the old downtown, and then below the overpass, or, immediately past the overpass, exit right on East Street, and then take the next right onto Carico Street. Both routes, after a little winding and precious few street signs, end up southbound on Jesse Hayes Road, which soon becomes Pioneer Drive. Take the right turn onto Kellner Canyon or Icehouse Canyon Road. At the fork, stay left on Icehouse Canyon Road, which is now also FR 112. About 1 mile past the national forest boundary, Icehouse CCC Recreation Area is on your left. Icehouse has vault toilets, picnic tables, horse hitches, and plenty of parking, but no water and no fees. Despite being labeled a campground on some maps, it is for day use only.

GPS Trailhead Coordinates	25 PINAL MOUNTAIN LOOP
UTM zone (WGS 84)	12S
Easting	518113.43
Northing	3688396.79
Latitude/Longitude	
North	33° 19' 64.5"
West	110° 48' 19.3"

SCENERY: ✿ ✿ ✿	DISTANCE: *9.45 miles*
TRAIL CONDITION: ✿ ✿	HIKING TIME: *5 hours*
CHILDREN: ✿	OUTSTANDING FEATURES: *The lookout tower*
DIFFICULTY: ✿ ✿ ✿	*on Aztec Peak, scenic overlooks, several biomes,*
SOLITUDE: ✿ ✿ ✿ ✿	*including burned forest in recovery*

This loop around the upper elevations of the Sierra Ancha Wilderness starts by climbing Aztec Peak to the Forest Service lookout tower via Abbey's Way. From the peak, it follows the service road down to Moody Point Trail and takes that path down the slope to its junction with Rim Trail. Going clockwise on Rim Trail reveals several biomes and takes you to overlooks of several deep gorges. The hike returns to high elevation via Parker Creek Trail, which terminates at the Carr trailhead. A brief stroll down the road takes you back to Abbey's Way trailhead. Many parts of this hike, particularly Rim Trail, have had substantial fire damage, which may make it unsuit-able for those with smaller legs.

🚶🚶 Abbey's Way Trail 151 starts to the right (north) side of the road, opposite the little parking area. The singletrack through the woods quickly crosses a little seep and then enters a meadow. Beyond the meadow are the remains of an apple orchard, part of the old Peterson Ranch for which this trail was once named.

Past the meadow, you first encounter the effects of the April 2007 Coon Fire. The large trees are all charred and waiting to fall over, but sapling and brush grow in profusion, often crowding the trail. This hasn't hurt the deer and elk population at all, as their scat is frequently encountered on the trail.

Within 1 mile, the trail starts climbing the actual peak via long switchbacks. Behind you, to the west, you have great views of Work-man Canyon, and to its south, Carr Peak. At about 1.65 miles, and 7,748 feet, you emerge at the top of Aztec Peak, a flat, grassy outcrop

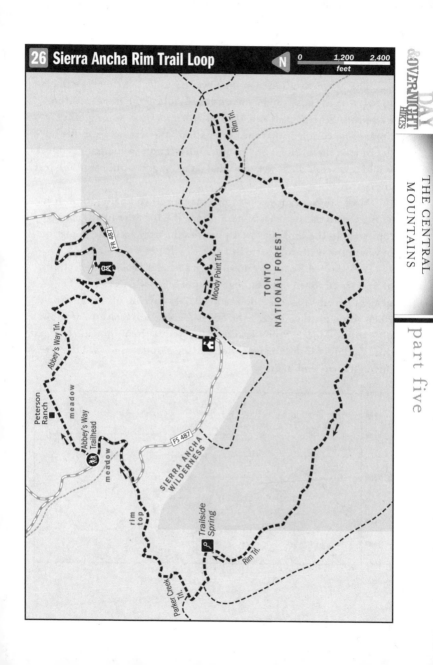

26 Sierra Ancha Rim Trail Loop

N   0   1,200   2,400
feet

DAY
&OVERNIGHT
HIKES

THE CENTRAL
MOUNTAINS

part five

FR 487

Abbey's Way Trl.

Peterson
Ranch

meadow

Abbey's Way
Trailhead

meadow

rim
top

Parker Creek Trl.

Moody Point Trl.

Rim Trl.

TONTO

NATIONAL FOREST

FS 487

SIERRA ANCHA
WILDERNESS

Trailside
Spring

Rim Trl.

decorated with a few ponderosa pine trees and the steel tower of the Forest Service lookout station.

The rangers stationed at the tower basically live there. In the late 1970s, one of those rangers was Edward Abbey, the famous author who wrote *Desert Solitude* and *The Monkey Wrench Gang,* among other works. The rumor is that the designation "151" comes from the bottles of rum the militant environmentalist (and unrepentant redneck) would toss from the tower, and that later rangers would find for years afterward.

Most rangers enjoy company, especially if you bring food. It is a long way to the store from here. Since the fire, the hand-marked topo map in the lookout tower provides the only accurate depiction of where the trails now actually run.

Take Forest Road 487 down from the peak. Pass some sections of unburned forest—just enough to appreciate what was lost. Go straight (south) past the side road (487A) spurring off to the ranch. Keep going until you reach the Forest Service workstation, at about 3.25 miles. Moody Point Trail 140 crosses the road immediately past this. Go left, off the roadway, descending east down toward the rim, through ferns and brush.

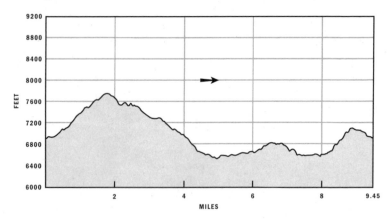

At about 4 miles, the trail starts switchbacking as you descend steeply into the drainage of Deep Creek. On the far side of that, the trail levels out a bit as the landscape shifts to scrub juniper and manzanita. Soon, Moody Point Trail will descend past its namesake and then into the deeper reaches of the Sierra Ancha, bottoming out at 3,000 feet on the banks of Cherry Creek. Long before that, though, it meets Rim Trail.

The signed junction with Rim Trail 139 marks the halfway point of the hike. Several boulders nearby provide a resting spot. When ready, head right, roughly south, down Rim Trail. The trail is rocky at first, but then eases up, at least the part beneath your boots. Soon you enter the boundaries of the Coon Fire. Dead trees blow over faster than the crews can clear them from the trail, and these will be a regular hazard. However, the absence of standing trees allows spectacular views of the canyon.

Between gorges, you often cross flat, grassy plains. Deer are frequently seen here, as are hawks. Near what the map describes as Armor Corral Springs, the trail disappears beneath a maze of fallen logs. The route goes uphill, and if in doubt, you can follow the little wash (easier on the far side) up the slope until you see the cairns again. It jogs uphill in a couple of legs into a stand of ponderosas as it winds back around the rim.

Back at the edge of the rim, you narrowly pass by a deep and marvelous gorge, and then cross behind a hill. Along here, the trail curves all the way around to the northwest, dropping into more burned forest with lots of little plants but precious little shade. All manner of insects and lizards scurry and flutter about the young, new biome.

The canyon below contains Coon Creek. Keep an eye out for a castle-like rock formation called The Palisades just past the 7-mile mark. At about 8 miles you pass Trailside Spring, identifiable only by the profusion of weeds in the drainage upslope of the trail. A quarter mile past this, Rim Trail terminates in a T-intersection with Parker

Creek Trail 160. Go right at this intersection, roughly northeast, and definitely uphill.

Parker Creek Trail charges up the hill with straightforward brutality. It is steep, rocky, exposed to the sun, crowded with thorns, and occasionally blocked by deadfall. The bright side is that it does not take long to reach the top, where you enter a lovely stand of oaks and locust. After less than 1 mile of this, you come to the Carr trailhead. From here, take the short jaunt down FR 487. Along the way, you'll round a meadow lined with aspen trees; soon after, you reach the Abbey's Way trailhead.

DIRECTIONS: From Globe, take AZ 188 north 14.5 miles, turn right on AZ 288 north, and continue 25 miles, crossing the Salt River and heading up the mountains. AZ 288 is only partially paved and still follows the same switchbacks up the mountain as the stagecoach route it was built to replace did, so don't plan on going any faster than 40 mph and, most of the way, slower than that. Pass the Sierra Ancha Research Station and Rose Creek Campground to turn right on FR 487 (near mile marker 284), a graded dirt road following Workman Creek several miles past two day-use areas and Falls Campground. If road conditions are poor, all vehicles may be stopped at the gate just above Falls Campground. If not, low-clearance vehicles will be obliged to stop at Workman Falls, about 0.5 miles farther down. Abbey's Way Trailhead, a dirt lot with no services, is less than 1 mile past the falls.

GPS Trailhead Coordinates	26 SIERRA ANCHA RIM TRAIL LOOP
UTM zone (WGS 84)	12S
Easting	507031.22
Northing	3741409.3
Latitude/Longitude	
North	33° 48' 46.3"
West	110° 55' 26.5"

Salome Wilderness

SCENERY: ✿ ✿ ✿	DISTANCE: *10.7 miles*
TRAIL CONDITION: ✿ ✿ ✿	HIKING TIME: *7 hours*
CHILDREN: ✿	OUTSTANDING FEATURES: *Big pink boulders,*
DIFFICULTY: ✿ ✿ ✿ ✿	*scenic overlooks, riparian swimming area, waterfalls*
SOLITUDE: ✿ ✿ ✿ ✿	

There are many places in Arizona named Hell's Hole (two are in the Tonto National Forest). This one, in the Salome Wilderness, is the most famous and accessible. That said, it remains relatively remote. This hike goes over a couple of ridges and then descends 1,000 feet into the canyon, near the confluence of Reynolds and Workman creeks. The hiking time allows for a slower pace up the switchbacks. Many hikers do this as an overnight.

🚶 Hell's Hole Trail 284 starts out as a remnant dirt road past a sign about how the Apache took care to leave no trace. What the sign doesn't mention is that this had more to do with military necessity than ecological concern. This road goes straight up and over a couple of hills through pine—oak forest. As it passes the buildings near the creek (a private ranch), the official trail becomes singletrack. It continues over and around the bluff then starts switchbacking sharply down into the creek. This is foreshadowing.

The creek is a lovely riparian area, and normally flowing. Grass, sycamores, and huge cottonwoods line its rocky banks. The path to climb out is about a hundred feet upstream of where the switchbacks dump you. Now you clamber over another pine-covered hill and into the Salome Wilderness. On the far side of the hill, you encounter a huge pink boulder balanced on a tree by the side of the trail. A dozen yards later, a seep puts out just enough water to muddy the track.

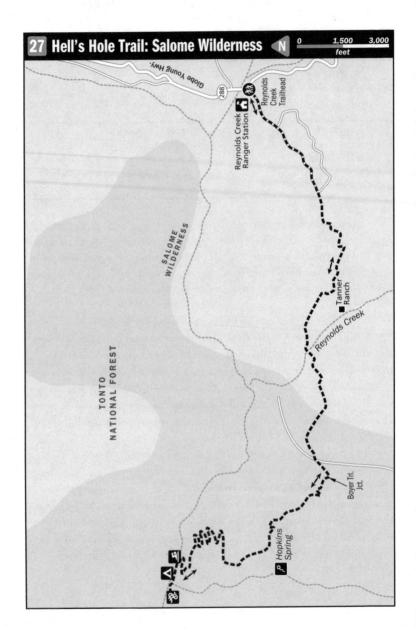

27 Hell's Hole Trail: Salome Wilderness

N

0   1,500   3,000
feet

Globe Young Hwy.

288

Reynolds Creek
Ranger Station

Reynolds Creek Trailhead

SALOME WILDERNESS

TONTO
NATIONAL FOREST

Tanner Ranch

Reynolds Creek

Boyer Trl. Jct.

Hopkins Spring

Keep climbing past that landmark until you reach the ridgetop.

The top is covered in transition scrub: juniper, oak, manzanita, and scrub oak. Once over the top, you quickly arrive at the junction with Boyer Trail. At 2.5 miles in, this is near the halfway point of the journey in. Boyer Trail goes south another 5 miles through the wilderness, passing several old homesteads. Stay right on Hell's Hole Trail.

As you make your way across the rocky and relatively exposed hilltop, keep an eye out for horned lizards, popularly called horny toads, especially in warm weather. The trail turns northwest for a little more than 1 mile as it crosses the ridgetop. At the north end, it starts switchbacking down into the enormous chasm that is opening before you. Those stark cliffs drop from 6,000 feet to 4,400 feet, and you will descend almost that distance on your side.

There will be 11 to 15 switchbacks, depending on where you start counting and how you define "switchback." Most of them are 400 to 600 feet long. They can be steep, rocky, overgrown, and thin, but rarely all four at the same time, and they often continue as an easy singletrack. The real challenge is mental—no matter how much you prepared for the hike, these things take longer than you expected.

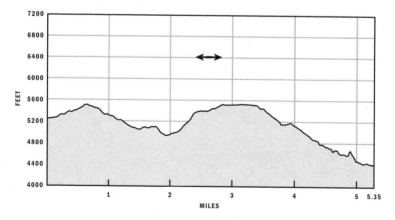

On your way down, you cross a pink granite rockslide. You also occasionally see other granite boulders or an enterprising ponderosa pine that has found a place to grow on the steep slope. Juniper and oak grow on the slope as well, but there are too few to provide consistent shade. Your most constant companion, though, will be scrub oak, which frequently crowds the trail.

The steeper switchbacks mean you're nearing the bottom, but you can see and hear the river at this point anyway. The trail flattens out at a large pool bordered by huge pink granite boulders. Just downstream of this, a narrow track leads you to a couple of established campsites. People have left firepits and broken shovels for your convenience.

The campsites, at 5.1 miles, indicate the end of the official trail. A trace route marked by cairns continues downstream, however, and is worth following. In less than 0.25 miles, you reach a high, narrow waterfall, where an uphill spring feeds the creek. At this point, the trail becomes more of a route, and you'll have to do a bit of scrambling to follow it to the small falls and big pools beyond.

Your hike out, though mostly uphill, will actually be a little easier (mentally) now that you know what you're in for with the switchbacks.

DIRECTIONS: From Globe, take AZ 188 north 14.5 miles, then turn right on AZ 288 north and continue 25 miles, across the Salt River and up the mountains. AZ 288 is only partially paved and still follows the same switchbacks up the mountain that the stage-coach route it was built to replace did, so don't plan on going any faster than 40 mph and, most of the way, slower than that. Pass the Sierra Ancha Research Station and, later, Rose Creek Campground to turn left at the pullout for Reynold's Group Site. The dirt road dead-ends at the trailhead, a dirt lot with no services, just past the campground.

GPS Trailhead Coordinates	27 HELL'S HOLE:
	SALOME WILDERNESS
UTMzone (WGS 84)	12S
Easting	503083
Northing	3747372.9
Latitude/Longitude	
North	33° 52' 17.0"
West	110° 58' 31.0"

SCENERY: ✿ ✿ ✿	DISTANCE: *10 miles*
TRAIL CONDITION: ✿ ✿ ✿	HIKING TIME: *7 hours*
CHILDREN: ✿	OUTSTANDING FEATURES: *Stunning canyon*
DIFFICULTY: ✿ ✿ ✿ ✿	*vistas, outstanding riparian swimming and*
SOLITUDE: ✿ ✿	*fishing holes*

This arduous but popular hike crosses several hills before climbing a ridge and then descending 1,800 feet into the Hell's Gate Wilderness and Hell's Gate itself: the steep canyon where Haigler Creek flows into Tonto Creek. The half mile immediately into or out of the canyon is notoriously steep; the hiking time reflects the difficulty of climbing back out. Although described here as a one-way car shuttle (though, admittedly, a monstrous car shuttle), this route is commonly done as an out-and-back from the north side, frequently as an overnight.

🚶🚶 The dirt road that leads from the trailhead crosses a maze of alternate roads and tracks all heading roughly south through the pine-covered hills. The true path is marked, if you look carefully, but any path that takes you south will likely get you there. You follow a barbed-wire fence to your left. The route will climb a hill, then descend into a drainage, where a seep keeps a patch of grass alive and perhaps pools into a hole full of black water.

After 1 mile, all the routes converge near a corral before the remnant road climbs steeply, at jeep-trail grade, to the top of a hill. From that point on, the path down into the canyon is a singletrack. The trail winds down the hill and across and down Apache Ridge, passing a cattle tank and, later, the wilderness boundary, at just past 4 miles.

As you descend, you will leave the pine forest for juniper—oak scrub. The trail winds a little to the east to follow Hell's Gate Ridge down toward the edge of the canyon. You encounter a few steep and

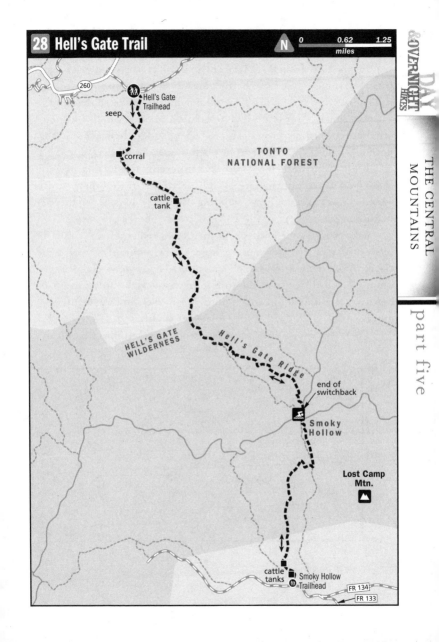

N

0   0.62   1.25
miles

Hell's Gate Trailhead

260

seep

corral

TONTO NATIONAL FOREST

cattle tank

HELL'S GATE WILDERNESS

Hell's Gate Ridge

end of switchback

Smoky Hollow

Lost Camp Mtn.

cattle tanks

Smoky Hollow Trailhead

FR 134

FR 133

rocky switchbacks, but these are merely short warm-ups for what is to come.

From the 7-mile mark (the last 0.5 miles), the switchbacks earn their fearsome reputation: being stairwell steep, exposed, and chock full of rock and scree. You'll spend much of that stretch stepping with the side of your boots in a desperate and occasionally futile attempt to not slide down the scree. Then, suddenly, you are in the boulder-strewn river bottom, just below 4,000 feet elevation.

Both Tonto and Haigler creeks are perennial. Fluctuating water levels have wiped out any formal trails across or around their confluence, so you're on your own hopping boulders and pushing through brush to get anywhere in this riparian oasis. The Tonto enters through a steep-walled canyon formed from red and brown cliffs and pauses to form a large swimming hole. Fish (frequently trout), swim about in the clear water, largely untroubled by anglers. Haigler's entrance, a little south of the end of the switchbacks, is less dramatic but still surrounded by cottonwoods, sycamores, and all the other greenery that comes with a constant water supply.

There are a few good campsites down here, but they fill quickly

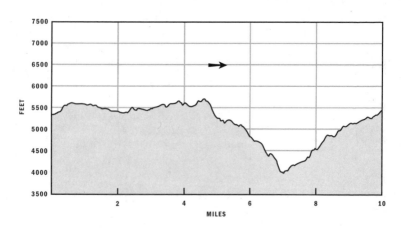

on weekends with good weather. On such weekends, you will certainly have company here. Make friends. Don't skinny-dip.

All of the above assumes low to normal water levels. At high water, the rivers silt up, the campsites are submerged, and crossing can be a cold and hazardous business.

The southern route out ascends Smoky Hollow, whose mouth is on the far side of Haigler Creek, just upstream (east) of the confluence. There is no established trail from the swimming hole; you'll have to dead-reckon across the wedge between the rivers. However, once you realize you need to be to the left of the large cliff south of the confluence, the route is easy to find.

The trail climbing the hollow crosses the seasonal drainage almost immediately and proceeds up the left (east) side of the canyon. This section is goat-trail narrow and very steep as you rapidly leave the creek bed below you. No switchbacks here—you march straight up the canyon.

The track levels out on a grassy juniper-bordered slope at about the 4,300-foot line. You will cruise that elevation toward a stand of oak, where the creek bed has risen to meet the trail. You pass a couple of campsites before you cross the creek bed, and then head down canyon and north 100 yards, following the cairns. There you encounter the remnant road, filled with all colors of rock, which will lead you out, starting with three stiff switchbacks.

These lead you to the top of a rising ridge covered in grassy transition scrub. The jeep trail goes mostly straight over the top of this ridge, with several steep climbs as you leave the canyon behind. At the end of the second climb, turn around and gaze upon Hell's Gate stretching out behind you in all its rugged glory. That's why you're tired.

You cross out of the wilderness boundary and then keep climbing. Soon you encounter a series of cattle tanks; cow trails start to wander around the roadway, masquerading, for the unwary, as hiking paths. Be selective about these, as cows have limited judgment. The true path is on the roadway.

Near the top of the ridge, the trail runs into Forest Road 133 at the Smoky Hollow trailhead, which consists of a patch of gravel and a wooden sign.

DIRECTIONS: Hell's Gate Trailhead: From Payson, take AZ 260 east, past Star Valley, toward Little Green Valley, a settlement and a speed-trap where the divided highway ends. Make the right onto FR 405A (the only exit in Little Green Valley). Stay on the dirt; all the paved portions are private driveway. The Hell's Gate trailhead will be less than 1 mile down the road on your right.

Smoky Hollow Trailhead: From Payson, take AZ 260 east 24 miles to FR 291 (graded dirt). Turn right and go 3 miles until your next right on FR 200. Take that road south, over numerous mountains, until its T-junction with AZ 288, north of Young. Turn right (south) toward Young. As you pass through Young, go straight where AZ 288 makes a left turn and continue west until you reach FR 129. At the fork in a couple of miles, stay right on FR 129. About 1 mile later, FR 133 heads left. Past this point you'll need a 4WD. Bounce the 8 miles winding up FR 133 to the trailhead on top of the ridge.

NOTE: Some published maps show incorrect forest road numbers. The road going up and around Fuller Mesa, properly designated FR 1673, is sometimes shown as FR 133 or FR 130. This is nothing more than a jeep trail, and while it can get you there, it is several colon-clenching miles out of your way.

While the shuttle route is just under 50 miles, very little of it is paved, and FR 133 will let you drive 10 mph, tops. Plan for a two-hour drive one way.

GPS Trailhead Coordinates	28 HELL'S GATE TRAIL
	HELL'S GATE TRAILHEAD
UTMzone (WGS 84)	12S
Easting	487366.89
Northing	3793137.13
Latitude/Longitude	
North	34° 16' 45.6"
West	111° 08' 14.1"

GPS Trailhead Coordinates	SMOKY HOLLOW TRAILHEAD
UTMzone (WGS 84)	12S
Easting	491128.14
Northing	3782534.31
Latitude/Longitude	
North	34° 11' 1.5"
West	111° 5' 46.6"

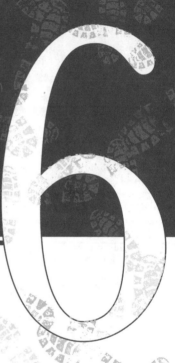

The
Mogollon
Rim

Explore
numerous
high peaks
deep gorges
babbling
river
beds
near-silent
deserts,
hundred-
year-old
mining
camps,
or thousand-
year-old
Native
American
settlements

SCENERY: ☆ ☆ ☆

TRAIL CONDITION: ☆ ☆ ☆

CHILDREN: ☆ ☆ ☆ ☆

DIFFICULTY: ☆ ☆ ☆

SOLITUDE: ☆ ☆

DISTANCE: *3.3 miles*

HIKING TIME: *2 hours*

OUTSTANDING FEATURES: *Springs, riparian area, abandoned and unfinished railroad tunnel*

The Colonel Devin Trail follows a historic route (now a utility route as well) up the face of the Mogollon Rim, along the banks of the East Verde River, crossing a couple of streams as it goes. The hike splits off near the top, along Railroad Trail, to visit an abandoned attempt to carve a train tunnel through the Rim. This popular, short hike is steep in places but still great for kids. The Colonel Devin portion is part of Arizona Trail, which runs across the state from Mexico to Utah.

Colonel Devin Trail 290 follows Highline Trail for about 100 feet from the Washington Park trailhead to a sign indicating that the dirt road going straight up the slopes is Devin Trail. (This road is still used as an access road for the local utility company.)

Colonel Thomas C. Devin, the trail's namesake, was a chief aid to General Crook in his campaign against the Apache in this area, and blazed the original route up this passage to the top of the Rim in 1869.

You climb up the slopes through spruce, oak, and pine that cover the foothills of the Rim. To your right, the East Verde River gushes continuously, but the road climbs away from it. To your left, every time you cross a gulley you will see the metal pipe of the aqueduct that also shares this route.

About 0.5 miles up, grass and ferns start to line the dirt road. You come a lot closer to the creek now, which babbles on a few feet from the roadway. All around you, you can see the escarpment. Devin Trail heads for a low point in the Rim. Higher portions tower above on either side. The road turns a little rougher and steeper as it

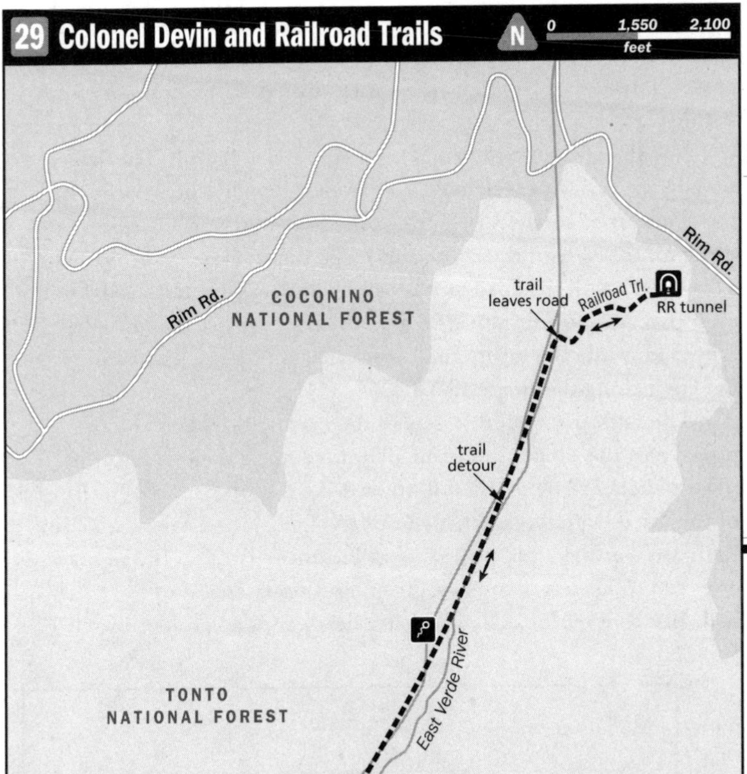

29 Colonel Devin and Railroad Trails
N
0
1,550
2,100
feet
Rim Rd.
Rim Rd.
COCONINO
NATIONAL FOREST
trail
leaves road
Railroad Trl.
RR tunnel
trail
detour
TONTO
NATIONAL FOREST
East Verde River
Pieper Hatchery
Springs
aqueduct
Houston Mesa Rd.
To
FR 32

climbs. Soon you encounter power lines to the left, and you cross a couple of streams where springs feed the creek. The creek itself supports a number of riparian trees, including Arizona sycamore and walnut.

Just shy of the 1-mile mark, you come to a detour. The "road" actually crosses the creek here, to run past Pieper Hatchery Springs, but a couple of singletracks, one going high and one going low, continue on this side of the creek and make for an easier journey. They will reunite with the road as it crosses back in about 100 yards. Soon after that, a sign will indicate where the trail crosses the now-dry creekbed, while the utility road continues on up the west bank. Take the right along the singletrack trail.

The rocky path winds through the granite boulders and the pines, past the remains of some primitive stone shelter. Soon, it starts switchbacking up the hill toward the top of the Rim. At the end of the third switchback, a little wooden sign indicates the cutoff for Railroad Tunnel Trail 390 (the trail number isn't on the sign). This goes east to make a torturous, steep, and rocky ascent of the creek bed. Just when it looks like the path dead-ends at a limestone cliff

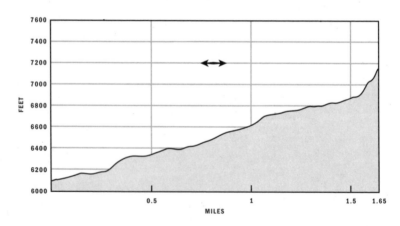

dripping with seep water, it crosses the drainage and climbs another few steep feet to the Railroad Tunnel site.

In the 1880s, James W. Eddy concocted a disastrously under-funded scheme to link Flagstaff and Globe via the Mineral Belt Railroad, part of which was to burrow through the mighty Mogollon Rim. Starting in 1883, men worked on and off until 1887, some being paid only in "stock," digging the tunnel that you will find on top of this little bluff. The remains of the powder house—another, larger building of stacked rock walls—still stands next to the tunnel, a 15-foot hole in the cliff that goes back about 70 feet into the Rim. Soft, damp sand covers the floor, while graffiti covers the walls.

The goat trail that seems to continue around the bluff to the west disintegrates after 100 yards, so return the way you came.

DIRECTIONS: From Payson, take AZ 87 north and turn right onto Forest Road 199, at the edge of town. If you reach Houston Mesa Campground, you've gone too far. Go slightly more than 10 miles north on this graded dirt road, past Freedom Acres and a couple of campgrounds, to Verde Glen and the Control Road FR 64. Turn left (west), and less than 1 mile later, turn right (north) onto FR 32. About 3 miles north of this, take FR 32A as it splits off to the right. This rough road goes another 2 miles, past numerous camp-sites, until it dead-ends at the trailhead. A high-clearance vehicle is needed for that last mile.

GPS Trailhead Coordinates	29 COLONEL DEVIN AND RAILROAD TRAILS
UTM zone (WGS 84)	12S
Easting	475988.89
Northing	3809946.24
Latitude/Longitude	
North	34° 25' 50.6"
West	111° 15' 40.8"

SCENERY: ☆ ☆ ☆	DISTANCE: *7.5 miles*
TRAIL CONDITION: ☆ ☆ ☆	HIKING TIME: *4 hours*
CHILDREN: ☆ ☆ ☆ ☆	OUTSTANDING FEATURES: *Scenic overlooks,*
DIFFICULTY: ☆ ☆ ☆	*rich riparian area, springs, best swimming hole in the*
SOLITUDE: ☆	*national forest*

This short and popular hike follows the old jeep trail down into the Fossil Springs Wilderness and to the wonderful riparian area and swimming hole fed by Fossil Springs, some of the most consistent springs in the area. Though the trailhead lies in the Tonto National Forest, the wilderness area does not. It is, however, absolutely worth crossing a line on the map (not to mention the elevation change) to get to it. The hiking time does not allow for playing in the water—for that, you'll want to leave yourself a couple of hours, if not a couple of days.

🚶 Fossil Springs Trail 18 starts at the sign-in station (where there is a logbook and a Forest Service pen). At that point, you can take either the roadway to the left or the steep, rocky shortcut trail to the right. The trail is tougher but a lot shorter. Go right and enter a level, gravel field dotted with a couple of lonely trees. On the far side of this, the route continues as a wide singletrack, rocky and relatively steep. This winds its way counterclockwise around and into the limestone canyon, through juniper and oak scrub that provides some greenery but little shade. The rocky and steep sections are generally short and are divided by moderate stretches of packed-dirt trail. The traffic is such that you'll always find a footpath that has been pounded to gravel on even the roughest section. The rocky prominence to the north is Nash Point.

About halfway down at the 2-mile mark, you pass a little campsite to the right that has an odd wooden structure beside a well-used fire pit. By the 3-mile mark, you have passed through a deer maze

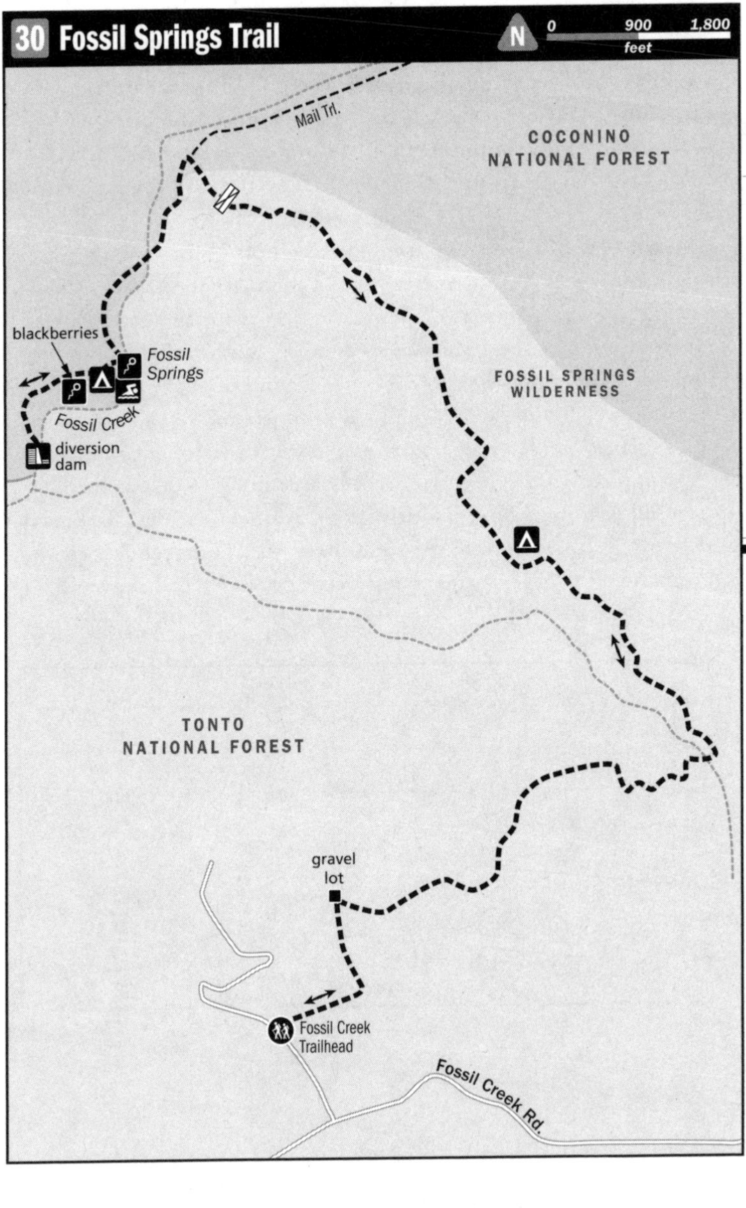

30 Fossil Springs Trail
N
0
900
1,800
feet
Mail Trl.
COCONINO NATIONAL FOREST
blackberries
Fossil Springs
Fossil Creek
diversion dam
FOSSIL SPRINGS WILDERNESS
TONTO NATIONAL FOREST
gravel lot
Fossil Creek Trailhead
Fossil Creek Rd.

and are approaching the T-junction with Mail Trail, which goes north (upstream), toward the western edge of the Mogollon Rim. Turn left (south), staying on Fossil Springs Trail, which quickly crosses the usually dry or nearly dry wash. Don't be discouraged; you're still uphill from the springs. Within 0.25 miles, brush and weeds will crowd the trail, and to your left, water runs through the creek.

At the base of a great elm tree, the first Fossil Spring feeds the creek through a 2-foot-diameter hole in the streambed that gushes water like a broken city main. This is the first of nine major springs (and countless seeps and burbles, depending on the water level) that pump out a combined 43 cubic feet per second of 72°F, mineral-heavy water year-round. A dozen yards downstream you can find several springs half this size before you reach the first big swimming hole, complete with a rope swing. The banks are crowded with ash, alder, and Arizona walnut, along with occasional boxelder, hackberry, and Arizona sycamore trees. Around these, wild grape, chokeberry, sumac, and all manner of ferns and weeds grow all along the bank.

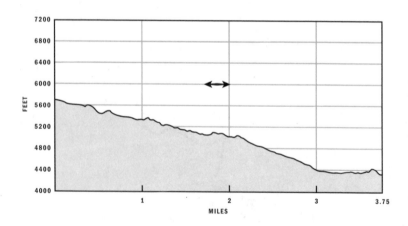

Fossil Springs are technically hot springs—72°F is a little warm for ordinary groundwater, though perfect for swimming. The most remarkable feature of the water, though, is the amount of calcium and bicarbonate it contains. As the creek flows downstream, these minerals settle on and eventually coat any object in the streambed—twigs, stones, garbage, and slow crayfish—giving them the fossilized appearance that lent the creek its name.

Up the right bank from the swimming hole, you will find some well-established campsites. This is a popular overnight destination both for backpackers and for groups of kids toting sleeping bags under their arms. These sites fill early on weekends. Past the campsites, the trail is choked with blackberries—a nonnative species that does well on this bank. Beside and beneath the blackberry canopy flows another big spring and several more seeps. Past the blackberries, the trail climbs a bluff, going 0.2 miles before descending again near the diversion dam. Behind the dam, predictably, lies a great, deep swimming hole. Beside it is another well-used campsite. This is the end of the hike, but not the end of the story.

For a hundred years, much of Fossil Creek's flow had been diverted by this dam, and one farther downstream, to run a pair of small hydroelectric power plants built in the early 1900s. Through the miraculous, and largely unprecedented, cooperative effort of the utility company and a consortium of environmental groups and government agencies, those power plants (which were functioning and profitable until the day they closed) are in the process of being dismantled, and the creek restored to its pre-1909 condition.

That's why Flume Trail, which runs south, downstream from this point, is closed to hikers; they are dismantling the flume it serviced right down to the bridges the trail crossed. As of summer 2008, they have yet to reach the concrete dam and the ladders around it, so the deep swimming hole just upstream will remain for a while.

As part of the restoration, fish biologists took some trouble to remove all the nonnative species from the creek (except for crayfish, which seem invincible) and restore the native species: desert chub, speckled dace, and Sonoran suckers. These are hardly high-profile game fish, but the wilderness area is closed to anglers nonetheless. The primary peril facing the new Fossil Creek is an old one: its popularity results in a lot of garbage. As you have probably already witnessed, not all of your fellow hikers have good judgment. Take some extra garbage out with you.

It is recommended that you treat any water you need; the upper reaches still drain through grazing lands.

Return the way you came.

DIRECTIONS: From Payson, take AZ 87 north about 17 miles, through Pine to the town of Strawberry. In Strawberry, turn left off the highway at the Strawberry Lodge to follow Fossil Creek Road (a.k.a. Forest Road 708) west through town and another 2 miles out past the town limits. The turnoff for the trailhead will be on your right, opposite FR 591. The trailhead can accommodate a dozen vehicles (though there will frequently be more than that). It has an outhouse and horse facilities but no water.

	30 FOSSIL SPRINGS TRAIL
GPS Trailhead Coordinates	
UTM zone (WGS 84)	12S
Easting	447759.75
Northing	3807508.26
Latitude/Longitude	
North	34° 24' 27.7"
West	111° 34' 06.3"

31 Oak Springs Trail

SCENERY: ✿ ✿ ✿	DISTANCE: *9 miles*
TRAIL CONDITION: ✿ ✿ ✿	HIKING TIME: *4.5 hours*
CHILDREN: ✿ ✿ ✿	OUTSTANDING FEATURES: *Scenic vistas of*
DIFFICULTY: ✿ ✿	*Strawberry Valley, Oak Springs*
SOLITUDE: ✿ ✿	

This shuttle hike allows you to eat lunch in Strawberry and then dinner in Pine while seeing some wonderful scenery in between. From just south of Strawberry, the trail follows the slope of Strawberry Mountain south toward Hardscrabble Road. Across the road, it merges with Trail 251, going down the canyon toward Oak Springs. Near the springs, the trail splits from 251, heading north over a couple of hills before crossing AZ 87 to reach the Pine trailhead. Parking on Hardscrabble Road makes for a shorter hike. This is part of the Arizona Trail, which runs from Mexico to Utah.

🥾 Oak Springs Trail 16 is the only trail originating from the obscure Strawberry trailhead. After crossing a limestone bluff, it descends sharply into a creek bed and travels a few hundred yards before climbing out, over red clay, up the slope of the ridge. Now you are in burned forest—the result of controlled burns—as witnessed by the numerous circles of charred timber. What remains of the pine and oak is healthy but somewhat spread out. Shade is only intermittent.

The trail proceeds along the north slope of Strawberry Mountain, between the 5,700- and 5,800-foot line, winding up and down around drainages, but presenting no serious elevation changes. It travels like a mini-golf version of the Highline Trail. This route is obviously popular with mountain bikers. Here and there a side road will intersect it to descend to one of the many cabins below you on the Rim. Stay on the trail. There are no signs along the path but many cairns, and in most places the packed-dirt track remains fairly obvious.

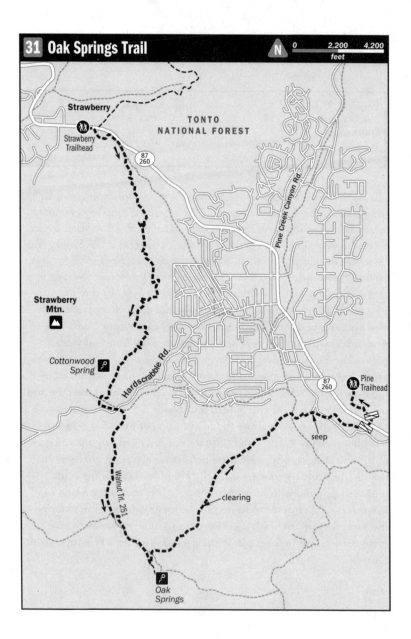

N

0   2,200   4,200
feet

Strawberry

Strawberry
Trailhead

TONTO
NATIONAL FOREST

87
260

Pine Creek Canyon Rd.

**Strawberry
Mtn.**

*Cottonwood
Spring*

Hardscrabble Rd.

87
260

Pine
Trailhead

seep

Walnut Trl. 251

clearing

*Oak
Springs*

For 3.5 miles the path goes like this, passing by pricey neighborhoods like Strawberry Hollow and the western slopes of Pine, which all lie down-slope from the trail. People pay big money so that hikers can look into their backyards, though, really, the huge cabins are mostly hidden by trees. Beyond, the Mogollon Rim towers over the mountain hamlets. Toward the southern end of the mountain, the trail starts winding down the slope, making the last descent over a series of switchbacks. At the 4-mile mark, it meets Hardscrabble Road, FR 428. Straight across the road, you will see the sign for Walnut Trail 251, the continuation of the hike.

You could park a shuttle vehicle here, cutting the hike in half, which might be most desirable if hiking with children. Much of the published material about this trail assumes starting or ending at Hardscrabble Road and focusing on the southern section with the actual spring.

To get there, follow Walnut Trail over the saddle and then down into the wash beyond. The trail stays close to the drainage as the wash deepens into a ravine and then a canyon. The forest turns greener and more lush as you descend. The trail crosses the creek

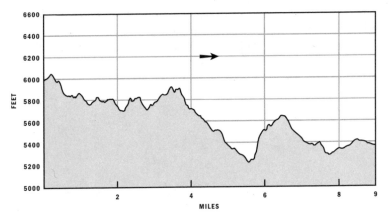

several times. A few crossings can involve cairn hunts, but with some attention these are easily managed. Within 2 miles you are walking through deep pine–oak forest.

At 2.5 miles, Oak Trail 16 splits from Walnut Trail 251. This is also the junction with Arizona Trail, which has reached this point coming northward on Walnut Trail. As a quick side trip, less than 0.25 miles farther down Walnut Trail, you will find Oak Springs, an excellent and reliable water source. Back at the junction, Oak Trail (and Arizona Trail) goes off to the left, turning sharply northeast. After crossing the creek, it then starts a long series of switchbacks up the slope of Oak Springs Canyon.

At the top of the hill, the track widens into a remnant jeep trail and descends straight down the slope (a river of brown rock). The transition juniper scrub on top of the hill gives way to shady pine and oak woodlands. This, in turn, gives way to sunnier controlled-burn remnants as you descend, making your way roughly northeast. You pass a grassy seep at the bottom of the hill.

Soon after, closely spaced fiberglass signs mark the road as it climbs over low hills and passes behind the backyards of Pine residents. Follow the signs along the road to the highway. You pass through gates on either side of the busy AZ 260/87, which obviously must be crossed with care. North of the highway, the trail crosses a drainage, climbs the small hill on the far side, and then follows the top of the hill where it briefly joins Highline Trail. From this point it is only a few hundred yards to the Pine trailhead.

DIRECTIONS: From Payson, take AZ 87/260 north about 13 miles toward Pine. Just before entering Pine, look for the Pine trailhead on your right. If you reach the Rimside Grill, you've passed it. The Strawberry trailhead is also just south of its namesake, which lies about 3 miles north of Pine, though no sign marks it. There is a slow vehicle turnout lane on the southbound side just south of the town limits. The dirt-road driveway to the trailhead is in the middle of that turnout lane.

GPS Trailhead Coordinates	31 OAK SPRINGS TRAIL
	STRAWBERRY TRAILHEAD
UTM zone (WGS 84)	12S
Easting	455512.31
Northing	3807320.18
Latitude/Longitude	
North	34° 24' 22.9"
West	111° 29' 2.6"

GPS Trailhead Coordinates	PINE TRAILHEAD
UTM zone (WGS 84)	12S
Easting	459241.89
Northing	3803730.05
Latitude/Longitude	
North	34° 22' 26.9"
West	111° 26' 35.9"

SCENERY: ☃ ☃ ☃ ☃	DISTANCE: *10 miles*
TRAIL CONDITION: ☃ ☃ ☃	HIKING TIME: *5 hours*
CHILDREN: ☃ ☃	OUTSTANDING FEATURES: *Riparian forest,*
DIFFICULTY: ☃ ☃ ☃	*springs*
SOLITUDE: ☃ ☃ ☃	

This hike follows Highline Trail briefly to Geronimo Trail, which goes over the foothills until it becomes East Webber Trail. The hike then follows East Webber Creek up the side of the Mogollon Rim to its source: two springs gushing from the rocks.

🚶 Cross the road from the trailhead, and then immediately cross Webber Creek onto Highline Trail 31. The Highline going west is a nice singletrack through the pine forest, punctuated with lava rock. Within 0.5 miles, you come to a junction marked by a sign and a huge alligator spruce tree. Take the right turn onto Geronimo Trail 240.

Geronimo Trail, for much of its course, consists of an orange jeep trail going up and down the hills through the pines and oak. At about 1.3 miles, though, watch for the singletrack shortcut going around the hill. This saves you from going over the hill like a jeep. The road skirts to the west of Camp Geronimo, a private youth camp. At 1.7 miles, watch for the spur road that dead-ends at the camp's gate. You need to stay west, taking a hard left around the bend.

Shy of the 2-mile mark, you come to the intersection with Milk Ranch Point Trail. Stay to the right, on Geronimo. You soon cross a stream and then come to the intersection with West Webber Trail, which goes to Turkey Springs and eventually Milk Ranch Point, on top of the Rim. The signs, made by youth from the camp, may be confusing. Stay straight on Geronimo Trail.

32 East Webber Creek Trail

N 0   1,700   3,400
feet

DAY &OVERNIGHT HIKES

THE MOGOLLON RIM

part six

COCONINO NATIONAL FOREST

Milk Ranch Point Rd.

Lee Johnson Spring

E. Webber Trl.

fallen log

Geronimo Trl. ends

TONTO NATIONAL FOREST

W. Webber Creek

Bear Spring

Camp Geronimo

Webber Creek

Highline Trl.

watch for singletrack

Geronimo Spring

Geronimo Trl.

Geronimo Trailhead

Webber Creek Rd.

FR 440

At 2.6 miles, the signs tell you that the dry creek you are crossing is West Webber Creek. After you cross West Webber Creek, you are in for a fairly sustained climb as the dirt road winds up and around the hill. At the top of the hill, the forest thins out and the trees get shorter, allowing you to see the Rim halfway up the sky to the north.

At 3.5 miles, Geronimo ends and the footpath of East Webber Trail 289 begins. Fallen logs block the road right before you get there. The dirt road heading to the right (west) leads to another gated entrance to Camp Geronimo. Across the road, burnt skeletons of trees with ferns all around them are evidence of previous fires. As you climb the hill, the road narrows to a singletrack through the woods.

Over the hill, where fires never reached, you drop into a fern-filled gulley shaded by oak and pine, where you will cross East Webber Creek. Past this crossing, the trail becomes a dusty romp through the pines until the next crossing, which features a huge fallen log. The trail continues climbing up the Rim, roughly parallel to the creek. You pull away to the left a bit and cross Patton Draw, a spring-fed tributary, before returning to the main creek, which you will closely follow the rest of the way up.

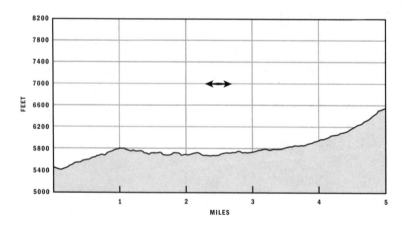

Fires have left the trees stripped of needles and leaves. Ravens above and around you add a haunting texture to the empty branches. Below, though, is plenty of green: ferns, wild grape, wolfberries, and, of course, occasional poison ivy.

The route is marked with yellow-tipped green stakes, but the trail would be easy to find even without them. Just past 4.5 miles, you cross the creek a third time. The trail past here gets steeper and rockier, winding its way around gray granite boulders covered with brown moss, through the low overgrowth of weeds, ferns, and sticker bushes. A half mile later, across the creek on the hillside to your left, you can see the big spring pouring through the rocks and ferns. Less than 0.25 miles farther, the second spring pours out over chocolate-colored rocks. Although the trail continues to the top of the Rim, it won't get any better than this. Return the way you came.

DIRECTIONS: **From Payson, take AZ 87 north approximately 12 miles and turn right on Forest Road 64, also known as Control Road. Take the graded, dirt Control Road 6 miles east to the left turn onto FR 440. The Geronimo trailhead is 2 miles up this road, just south of the gate to Camp Geronimo. The patch of gravel can accommodate three vehicles and has no services other than informative signs.**

GPS Trailhead Coordinates	32 EAST WEBBER CREEK TRAIL
UTM zone (WGS 84)	12S
Easting	466401
Northing	3806655.43
Latitude/Longitude	
North	34° 24' 2.8"
West	111° 21' 56.0"

33 Horton Springs Loop

SCENERY: ✿ ✿ ✿ ✿	DISTANCE: *9.5 miles*
TRAIL CONDITION: ✿ ✿ ✿	HIKING TIME: *6.5 hours*
CHILDREN: ✿ ✿ ✿	OUTSTANDING FEATURES: *Rim vistas, gushing*
DIFFICULTY: ✿ ✿ ✿	*spring, riparian meadows, wildlife*
SOLITUDE: ✿ ✿ ✿ / ✿ ✿	
(Derrick/Horton)	

This popular loop travels up the Mogollon Rim to the always gushing Horton Springs, using Highline Trail 31 to connect Derrick Trail 33 and Horton Creek Trail 285. The Rim's transition forest and Horton Creek's riparian channel support a wide variety of flora and fauna, from agave cacti to ponderosa pine and butterflies to mule deer.

If you have young children or smaller dogs, you may want to just take the easiest portion of the route out and back along Horton Creek Trail. Both trails are popular with equestrians, and trail etiquette suggests that hikers yield to horses.

🚶🚶 Walk past the Horton Creek trailhead near the campground entrance and continue forward to locate the Derrick trailhead, which is well inside Upper Tonto Creek Campground, past the restrooms. Look for a big log lying on the side of the hill. The trail passes alongside the log, which is easier to locate than the trailhead sign at the bottom of the hill.

The trail starts south, up the hill, passes the log, and then turns eastward at the top of the hill. From there, follow the ridgeline up the Rim, through a well-integrated transition forest of pine, juniper, oak, manzanita (ironwood), and even Perry's agave and prickly pear cacti, all living together in peace. This trail sees far fewer travelers than Horton Trail, and you may be breaking spider webs with your face.

After 1 mile or so, a sign announces Derrick Spur Trail, which wanders overland down the slopes towards Kohl's Ranch. Stay on the main trail heading east and up—always up. The trail is well defined

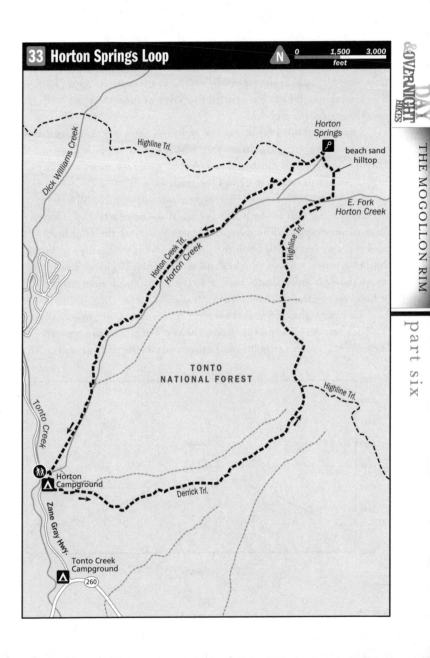

N   0   1,500   3,000
feet

Horton Springs

beach sand hilltop

Dick Williams Creek

Highline Trl.

E. Fork Horton Creek

Horton Creek Trl.

Horton Creek

Highline Trl.

Highline Trl.

TONTO NATIONAL FOREST

Tonto Creek

Horton Campground

Derrick Trl.

Zane Gray Hwy.

Tonto Creek Campground

260

but not without its difficulties. The wind, the lightning, the slope, and the condition of the soil often conspire to fell trees. Several trees lay across Derrick Trail, especially on the more exposed upper half. The trail through here has eroded to a river of football-sized, red, sparkling sandstone rocks.

The barbed-wire fence to your right indicates less than 0.5 miles to the junction with Highline Trail, which will, in turn, lead to Horton Springs and Horton Trail. As you progress, more and bigger manzanita starts to crowd the trail.

Look for the sign marking the junction with the Highline lying on the ground next to the post to which it was once attached. Go left here (following the white diamond blazes that mark the Highline) and more or less uphill from the junction. Built originally as a horse trail to connect various ranches and settlements, Highline Trail runs more than 50 miles along the face of the Rim. You'll hike 3 miles of it between the Derrick and Horton trails.

To your right, the pine-covered Promontory Butte towers above. To your left, in between the pines, the vast expanse of the central Arizona high plains spreads out before you. In the near distance, AZ

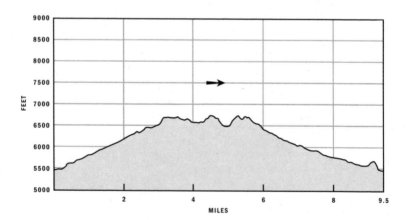

260 cuts across the hills north of Payson. Beyond that, look for the Green Valley Hills and, on a clear day, the Sierra Ancha Mountains.

While the Highline is fairly level across its length, this section has several steep climbs and descents of a few hundred feet. With each hill you go up and down, pine and oak crowd out more of the transition flora. By the time you descend into the ravine of the East Fork of Horton Creek, the sandstone has yielded to lichen-covered granite, and the pine trees are firmly in control of the neighborhood.

The East Fork of the Horton is usually dry, but during spring, or after heavy rain, you may have to wade across it. Grass and ferns line the trail through here, making for a pleasant spot to catch your breath before the last big climb of this loop—the Highline switchbacks steeply out of this ravine. On top of the hill, you'll find soft, white sand, as if from a beach; this is one of the few really good camping spots on the Highline.

The next long descent goes to the West Fork of Horton Creek, which flows constantly at this elevation. You can use one of several combinations of rocks and logs to cross the stream, but all of them are slippery; be careful. Once across, look for a gated fence, an open dirt area, and some stupendously large maple and fir trees. This spot is popular with picnickers and day-hikers. If you scramble 100 yards up the hill, you'll find the springs rushing out from beneath a pile of boulders with enough pressure to force you to shout if you attempt conversation. If you should bear a little left, through the cattle maze, the trail continues (arduously) to the top of the Rim.

A little trail leads down the side of the stream, but do not be fooled; it dead-ends in a couple hundred yards. The Horton Creek trail junction lies a bit farther west on the Highline, literally around the next bend. A sign points out a decaying wagon road plunging downhill. The upper third of the Horton is littered with the same sparkling sandstone rocks that vexed your footing on the Derrick, but the trail is less frequently blocked by logs and far more frequently traveled. Instead of spider webs, though, look out for horse apples.

A huge pile of granite boulders means you're getting near the creek again, and grass and ferns have pushed aside the dusty pine needles. To your left, Horton Creek tumbles noisily over a number of boulder falls on its way down the Rim. Riparian vegetation, cottonwoods, wild grapes, and a fair amount of poison ivy cover the banks. The trail wanders away from the creek and takes you along another old wagon road. Soon you'll come to a sizable rock cairn, where you must choose the old wagon road or a footpath.

The footpath (on your left), winds up and down the side of the creek and then wanders across a grassy plain. The old wagon road just descends through the pines. They intersect in 0.5 miles. By this time, unless overwhelmed by rain or snowmelt, the thirsty soil will have sucked Horton Creek dry. A quarter mile down you will cross its bone-dry boulder field of a creek bed to reach the trailhead at the entrance to the campground.

DIRECTIONS: Take AZ 260 to the Tonto Creek Recreation Area turn-off (Forest Road 289), about 16 miles north of Payson. Follow FR 289 north for about 1 mile to the Upper Tonto Creek Campground. Drive past this (unless you plan to camp there), cross the bridge, and park in the picnic area. Walk back across the bridge (which crosses the perennially flowing Tonto Creek) 200 yards to the campground.

Both the picnic area and the campground have vault toilets, and the campground has water. Fees for the concession-hosted campground are $13 per vehicle per night. Tonto Creek is popular with trout fishermen.

GPS Trailhead Coordinates	33 HORTON SPRINGS LOOP
UTM zone (WGS 84)	12S
Easting	0491364.2
Northing	3799595.7
Latitude/Longitude	
North	34° 22' 21"
West	111° 05' 40.0"

34 Highline Trail: *Washington Park to Geronimo*

SCENERY: ✿ ✿ ✿	DISTANCE: *9.4 miles*
TRAIL CONDITION: ✿ ✿ ✿	HIKING TIME: *5 hours*
CHILDREN: ✿ ✿	OUTSTANDING FEATURES: *Various vegetation*
DIFFICULTY: ✿ ✿ ✿	*zones, springs and creeks, ghost forests, panoramic*
SOLITUDE: ✿ ✿ ✿	*views*

This car-shuttle hike follows a section of Highline Trail from Washington Park to Camp Geronimo along the western third of the Mogollon Rim escarpment. From Washington Park, the hike goes west over the foothills and along the slope of the Rim, hovering at around the 6,100-foot line and crossing several creeks and springs as it goes. It also crosses the burned remains of the 1990 Dude Fire before finally heading south and downhill toward the Geronimo trailhead. This segment of the Highline is also part of Arizona Trail, which runs across the state from Mexico to Utah.

🚶🚶 Highline Trail 31 was originally blazed to link various ranches and homesteads along the Mogollon Rim. It runs 51 miles all told, across six designated trailheads.

A hundred yards past the trailhead, you come to a signed intersection with dirt-road Colonel Devin Trail. Stay on the singletrack trail heading left (west). In less than 0.25 miles, you will encounter another utility road. Again, stay straight on the trail. The path is lined with red sandstone and sparkling basalt as it wanders through oak, pine, and spruce forest interspersed with manzanita and sugarberry brush.

At the 0.8-mile mark, you come to a private ranch road near where it fords a little stream. Follow the road across the stream; take the singletrack through ferns and up the hill again. Keep straight (west) and you'll see the white diamond blaze of Highline Trail marking your exit from the road.

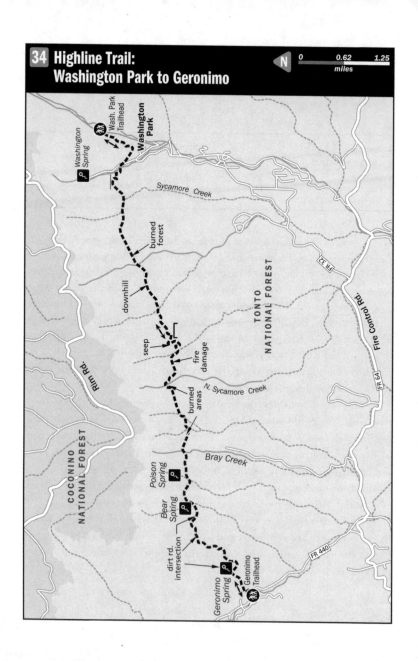

N

0   0.62   1.25
miles

Wash. Park Trailhead

Washington Park

Washington Spring

Sycamore Creek

burned forest

downhill

seep

fire damage

N. Sycamore Creek

burned areas

TONTO

NATIONAL FOREST

FR 32

Fire Control Rd.

FR 64

Rim Rd.

COCONINO

NATIONAL FOREST

Bray Creek

Poison Spring

Bear Spring

dirt rd. intersection

Geronimo Spring

Geronimo Trailhead

FR 440

On top of that ridge, about 1 mile in, you walk alongside a barbed-wire fence marked "no trespassing." That fence is not continuous, however; it dead-ends in a couple hundred yards, where it is wrapped to a tree, so that any human or beast could just stroll around to the other side. Its presence seems more of a political statement than an effective barrier. Past the fence, you climb up and down the foothills below the Rim, which hovers at about 6,100 feet. Ferns and grass grow up around the pines and oak, which takes some of the misery out of the many little climbs and descents.

At 1.7 miles, you cross Sycamore Creek, a lush belt of greenery and water running through the dusty pines. Past the creek, the trail climbs steeply. To your left, you have a pretty good view of the upper reaches of the Rim, Miller Point, Hi View Point, and what used to be a forest crowning it before fire reduced it to a collection of charred stumps. The trail tops out on a plateau covered by widely spaced oaks. But you soon descend back into the pines to reach a rough and rocky ravine crossing. On the far side of this ravine, you encounter your first stretch of the bare, burnt-orange sandstone, which you will see from time to time on this hike.

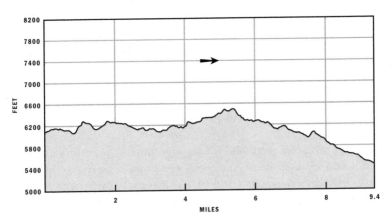

This path leads into the ruined forest, a victim of the 1990 Dude Fire. Twenty-foot-tall stumps, blackened by flames, line the field like an arboreal cemetery. The tops of these trees all fell here, but someone took the trouble to clear them from the trail.

Just past 3 miles, you must head down the red sandstone wash instead of crossing it the way you did other washes and drainages. Follow the cairns down the hill to about the 6,000-foot line, and then head west again. The trail past here is an easy singletrack through large alligator junipers and occasional patches of sandstone. Right at the 4-mile mark, someone made a little bench and placed it trailside. Take a rest, because after this you climb steeply, passing a seeping little spring before climbing to the top of the ridge.

You then descend down into and across a ravine to emerge in a clearing made by fire. The trail is faint through here, but just keep straight, heading west by southwest, and you will see cairns soon enough. A second even more charred field waits across the gulley. Once you cross that—following the cairns, for the track is faint—you come to some ferns and North Sycamore Creek, identified by a little wooden sign.

Climb out through the ferns and then start winding along the ridge and through the forest of charred trees, and you can see the panorama of the Tonto Basin that makes this trail famous. Past the lower ridgelines of Diamond Point and Houston Mesa tower the Mazatzal Mountains.

On the far side of the clearing, you cross a limestone-lined ravine. This crossing has been washed out a few times and will baffle the unwary. You may have to go downstream 100 yards or so to find a way back up.

Past this creek scramble, you traverse more brick-colored sandstone and scrub juniper, then encounter a spooky patch where the trees have been charred to cinders. But that clears the view ahead to see the rocky prominences of the Mogollon Rim, specifically Milk

Ranch Point, a peninsular outcropping from the escarpment.

At about 5.6 miles, you cross Bray Creek. As you cross, you can clearly see who won the contest for tallest cairn. Now you have returned to living pine forest, with needles on the trees and grass on the ground.

Past the 7.25-mile mark, you will encounter the first of two unmarked jeep roads. Stay on the trail as it starts turning south in a long series of switchbacks down the ridge. At first the switchbacks seem to wander through the lava rocks haphazardly. The grade is gentle, but there are many stumble-rocks and seemingly random turns. As you descend, they stretch out, and the trail itself becomes more orderly.

At the 9-mile mark, you briefly follow a jeep trail across the stream. Less than 100 yards past that, up the hill, the trail breaks off into a singletrack again. This track continues long, gently graded switchbacks heading south and downhill until finally emerging at the Geronimo trailhead.

DIRECTIONS: Washington Park Trailhead: From Payson, take AZ 87 north, and turn right onto Forest Road 199 at the edge of town. If you reach Houston Mesa Campground, you've gone too far. Go just more than 10 miles north on this graded dirt road, past Freedom Acres and a couple of campgrounds, to Verde Glen and Control Road, FR 64. Turn left (west), and then, in less than 1 mile, turn right (north) onto FR 32. About 3 miles north, take FR 32A as it splits off to the right. This rough road goes another 2 miles, past numerous campsites until it dead-ends at the trailhead. A high-clearance vehicle is needed for that last mile.

Geronimo Trailhead: From Payson, take AZ 87 north approximately 12 miles and turn right on FR 64 (Control Road). Take the graded dirt Control Road 6 miles east until you turn left on FR 440. The Geronimo trailhead is 2 miles up this road, just south of the gate to Camp Geronimo. The patch of gravel can accommodate three vehicles and has no services other than informative signs.

Of course, the easiest way to get from one trailhead to the other is via FR 64, on which the junction with FR 440 lies about 4.5 miles west of the junction with FR 32, for a total shuttle distance of around 12 miles.

GPS Trailhead Coordinates	34 HIGHLINE TRAIL:
	WASHINGTON PARK TO GERONIMO
	WASHINGTON PARK TRAILHEAD
UTM zone (WGS 84)	12S
Easting	475988.89
Northing	3809946.24
Latitude/Longitude	
North	34° 25' 50.6"
West	111° 15' 40.8"

GPS Trailhead Coordinates	GERONIMO TRAILHEAD
UTM zone (WGS 84)	12S
Easting	466401
Northing	3806655.43
Latitude/Longitude	
North	34° 24' 2.8"
West	111° 21' 56.0"

Index

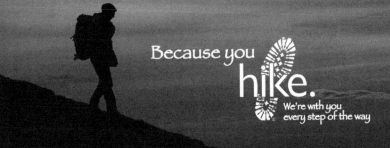

AMERICAN HIKING SOCIETY

Because you hike.

We're with you every step of the way

American Hiking Society gives voice to the more than 75 million Americans who hike and is the only national organization that promotes and protects foot trails, the natural areas that surround them and the hiking experience. Our work is inspiring and challenging, and is built on three pillars:

Volunteerism and Stewardship: We organize and coordinate nationally recognized programs – including Volunteer Vacations, National Trails Day® and the National Trails Fund –that help keep our trails open, safe and enjoyable.

Policy and Advocacy: We work with Congress and federal agencies to ensure funding for trails, the preservation of natural areas, and the protection of the hiking experience.

Outreach and Education: We expand and support the national constituency of hikers through outreach and education as well as partnerships with other recreation and conservation organizations.

Join us in our efforts. Become an American Hiking Society member today!

American Hiking Society

1422 Fenwick Lane · Silver Spring, MD 20910 · (301) 565-6704
www.AmericanHiking.org · info@AmericanHiking.org

DEAR CUSTOMERS AND FRIENDS,

SUPPORTING YOUR INTEREST IN OUTDOOR ADVENTURE, travel, and an active lifestyle is central to our operations, from the authors we choose to the locations we detail to the way we design our books. Menasha Ridge Press was incorporated in 1982 by a group of veteran outdoorsmen and professional outfitters. For 25 years now, we've specialized in creating books that benefit the outdoors enthusiast.

Almost immediately, Menasha Ridge Press earned a reputation for revolutionizing outdoors- and travel-guidebook publishing. For such activities as canoeing, kayaking, hiking, backpacking, and mountain biking, we established new standards of quality that transformed the whole genre, resulting in outdoor-recreation guides of great sophistication and solid content. Menasha Ridge continues to be outdoor publishing's greatest innovator.

The folks at Menasha Ridge Press are as at home on a white-water river or mountain trail as they are editing a manuscript. The books we build for you are the best they can be, because we're responding to your needs. Plus, we use and depend on them ourselves.

We look forward to seeing you on the river or the trail. If you'd like to contact us directly, join in at www.trekalong.com or visit us at www.menasharidge.com. We thank you for your interest in our books and the natural world around us all.

SAFE TRAVELS,

Bob Sehlinger

BOB SEHLINGER
PUBLISHER